Catherine and Neil Mackwood

HOW TO
SHAPE UP YOUR MAN

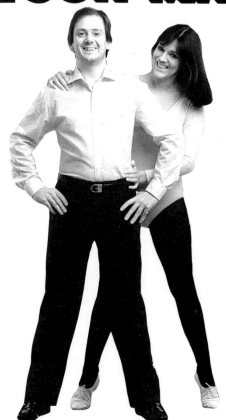

SPHERE

Sphere Books Limited
London and Sydney

This book is dedicated to
The Bodyworkshop School of Fitness and Health

Text © Catherine and Neil Mackwood 1986
Design © Shuckburgh Reynolds Ltd 1986

Produced and designed by Shuckburgh Reynolds Limited
289 Westbourne Grove, London W11 2QA

First published in Great Britain
by Sphere Books Limited 1986
30-32 Gray's Inn Road, London WC1X 8JL

ISBN 0 7221 5816 5

Photography by Christopher Cormack

Designed by Roger Pring

Charts of food fats reproduced
by kind permission of the Health Education Council.

Typesetting by SX Composing Ltd, Rayleigh, Essex

Printed in Portugal by Printer Portuguesa

Acknowledgments

Our special thanks to Tony Lycholat, sports
scientist and fitness adviser to The Bodyworkshop,
who was an active consultant on this book together
with physiotherapist Vivian Grisogono, who
helped so much on the fitness programme; to Dr
Craig Sharp, co-director of the Human Motor
Performance Laboratory, University of
Birmingham, who kindly allowed tests to be done
at the laboratory and completed the report while in
the midst of a busy schedule; to Dr Chandra Patel,
authority on stress management, who helped with
the stress section of the book; to Barbara Dale,
director of The Bodyworkshop School of Fitness
and Health, who teaches a balanced approach to
fitness which formed the basis of this book, and
finally to Dr Jan De Winter who helped initiate the
shaping up your man programme.

And a warm thank you to Hetty Einzig, Sophie
Warner and Nick Prest, who were supportive
companions to Neil on his journey
to meet his old self.

HOW TO
SHAPE UP
YOUR MAN

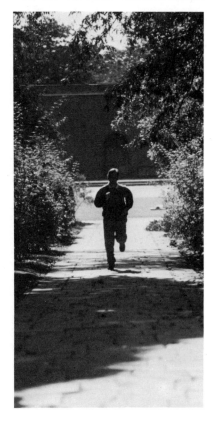

Contents

With a running commentary by Neil Mackwood

Introduction

The reason you picked up this book is probably the title and you are wondering – is it yet another trendy, unrealistic exercise book-cum-dieting manual? Obviously I'm biased but this book came about from a very real need. Neil wanted (or should I say needed?) to get into shape and we were both intrigued to see if we could find a way to get fit that wasn't fanatical, boring, time-consuming or painful. Working on the principle that life was far too short to become obsessed with health and fitness, we thought that there must be a middle way – a path through the jungle of often conflicting views on how to be healthy.

Let me start at the beginning. Neil seemed to spend the first three years of our marriage complaining about tiredness, even after a good night's sleep. Most mornings he felt and looked less than 100 per cent – more like 50 per cent. He was overweight (obese, as you will see later) and overworked, and he became more and more lethargic. Naturally, this affected his enjoyment of life, to the point of his simply not having the energy even to read a book. At the same time I was teaching at the Bodyworkshop where the women in my exercise classes kept asking me for ideas on how to get their husbands or partners into shape without hindering their enjoyment of life or taking up too much of their time. The idea of this book was emerging.

Unfortunately, the less fit you become, the less likely you are to do anything about getting fit and the harder you find it to move towards a healthier life-style. The process of becoming unfit is insidious. The victim completely adjusts to it until it has him by the throat and he finds himself gasping at the top of the stairs on the way to the annual medical. And the less fit you become, the less aware you are of good health. That's why the observer is often the best judge of fitness, and that is why we decided to aim this book at women and face the wrath of every feminist in the country. As the concerned observer you can see your partner's often almost imperceptible deterioration of fitness over the years, the changes due to stress, his job or lack of it, his sedentary life-style, his food and alcohol consumption. As his girth expands, so do your worries as you watch him become accustomed to tiredness, obesity, anxiety, as a normal way of life. To cope, he simply does less in order not to increase his tiredness, eats more to give himself more energy, drinks and smokes either to pep himself up or calm himself down depending on his needs.

Shaping Neil up was made easier by the fact that we were working to the same end. The three-month plan was a staggering success – a 25 per cent improvement in fitness, scientifically proved after extensive before and after tests at Birmingham University Sports Laboratories. Believe me – if Neil can do it, your man can too.

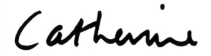

PS For proof of Neil's achievement, see the reports on pages 92-5 from Dr Craig Sharp, co-director of the Physical Education and Sports Science Department at Birmingham University, and from physiotherapist and sports specialist Vivian Grisogono.

Introduction

OK – the truth. I wasn't feeling exactly wonderful, nor was I feeling quite awful, but each morning I awoke with a soggy attitude and I swear it wasn't the alcohol. The time came one morning when Catherine's voice reached me distantly through the fog, suggesting that maybe it would not be such a bad idea, seeing how I looked and how I was feeling, for me to get into shape. "I'll make it easy. It will be fun. You won't have to give everything up – and you won't have to go up to a size 34 waist for your next suit," said the foggy voice.

What came to pass is recorded in this book. I admit that I was possibly the worst candidate for the venture or possibly, depending on your viewpoint, a pre-eminently suitable one. My life-style, you see, is based on the pursuit of information from people who keep company with the higher-profile politicians, the better-selling rock groups, the household faces of television and those familiar outrageous actors who have more dramas in their private lives than they ever present for public consumption on the stage. I am a journalist and we need to put ourselves about a bit.

That means calorific expense-account lunches, more calorific luncheons where no solids are consumed and yet more wonderfully unhealthy functions provided by publishers, club owners and the socially ambitious. Fun it is but it takes its toll, as one key figure in my conversion was quick to point out. "You can do just about anything to your body up to the age of 30 and then the creditors begin to gather and the bank account had better not be empty."

When that comment was made I might have heard a faint knock at the door – not that I was going to admit it – no doctor was going to startle me into a course of action I did not want to take. But for the sake of the marriage (OK, for my own good) I found myself implicated in a three-month regime the like of which I had not seen since school. But no enforced runs, compulsory swims in Icelandic pools or muscle-withering circuit training for me. I was to embrace something called the "Pleasure Principle" – strange, because that's exactly what I thought I had been doing all along.

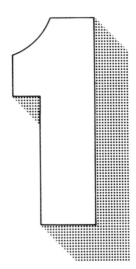

Gentle Persuasion

YOUR FIRST JOB is to persuade your man to get fit. This is no easy task. You obviously think he needs to be shaped up but he may be quite content as he is. He has probably become accustomed to his shape, his life-style, the way he feels. However anxious you are, never nag him. What is called for is the art of gentle persuasion. It is important to make him realise that, if our 12-week programme is adopted with the right attitude, getting fit need not be enormously time-consuming, nor need it detract from his pleasurable life-style. We have proved that.

Remember that there are no instant solutions and no need for you to panic your man into frenetic action. Remember too that everything here can apply as much to you as to him; the programme works equally well for women as for men. Its aim is to re-educate the system back to health with exercise that suits the individual's physical capacity, with a careful but still enjoyable diet and by learning to relax when overtired and overstressed. This will be achieved only by progressing gently. As the unfit man becomes fitter, he will have increasing respect for his body's machinery and will be less likely to continue with a damaging life-style as he feels the benefits brought to his life:

1 **More energy** With exercise, the body becomes more efficient so that simple everyday tasks become less tiring, and demanding work can be done without stiffness or fatigue.

2 **Less stress** The relaxation, both physiological and psychological, brought about by exercise reduces mental strain and promotes the health of the whole system.

3 **Fewer aches and pains** Regular activity improves muscle tone and muscular strength, preventing many postural problems that occur as a result of inactivity.

4 **Fewer illnesses** The body becomes more able to resist infection and recovers faster.

5 **Better looks** The body will have a better shape. Skin, eyes and hair will be in better condition, making him look good and feel good, and dramatically improving self-esteem.

6 **Better sex life** Believe it or not but active people are said to have better sex lives.

Your man's body

Begin by facing reality. There is no point in trying to mould a man into a shape that he basically isn't; apart from the fact that it won't work, it might also damage his health. Not all men can be he-men – and would you seriously want him to be? Underneath every bulging shirt there is not a long, lean Sebastian Coe waiting to emerge at the end of an intensive running programme. Nor is running a suitable exercise for everyone, even though, with the ever-increasing popularity of marathons, you might be led to believe that it was the only way to get fit.

Knowing about the three basic body types helps to determine what kind of shaping-up programme is likely to be most suitable – and therefore pleasurable – for your man. The physique classification system, worked out by American psychologist W. H. Sheldon, is not absolute. A man is classed as an ectomorph, mesomorph or endomorph according to whether his build is more characteristic of one type than the other two types.

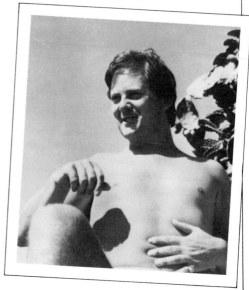

"I'm definitely the muscular, strong and altogether rather sportive type – but perhaps a little on the chubby side?"

Straight up and down
Ectomorphs are straight up and down in build, with narrow shoulders and hips, and long, thin arms and legs. They have little body fat and little muscle, and do not gain weight easily. Although losing weight is rarely a problem for ectomorphs, they often have poor muscular strength and their health will benefit considerably from a suitable exercise programme and a well-balanced diet. During prolonged strenuous exercise, their large skin surface and large nervous system help to speed up heat loss and prevent the build-up of internal body heat that leads to exhaustion, giving them high reserves of stamina. This makes them generally suited to exercises such as running and jogging, which require endurance, rather than to activities that demand bursts of speed.

Broad-chested and muscular
Men of the mesomorph type are muscular, with broad chests and shoulders, narrow hips and muscular arms and legs. They are generally strong and energetic, with little body fat and an ability to develop muscles easily, though if these are not used, their bodies are liable to run to fat.

The mesomorph makes a good all-round athlete, so men of this type are likely to be suited to any form of exercise, though they tend to be especially good at activities demanding strength and bursts of power, such as cycling.

Stocky and rounded
Endomorphs tend to have rounded bodies, even when not carrying extra weight, with rather short arms and legs that are fat around the upper arms and thighs and slender around the wrists and ankles. They normally carry quite a lot of body fat and are prone to put on weight easily. Because of their stocky build, they may appear deceptively strong and muscular. Exercise is particularly important for the endomorph. If, as is probable, he is overweight, an exercise such as swimming or cycling is likely to be suitable because no strain is placed on the weight-bearing joints of the body. Endomorphs often make good swimmers because their extra body fat helps protect them against the cold and give them buoyancy. Until he has lost some weight, he is unlikely to enjoy running or jogging, though brisk walking may be a good alternative.

❝If one of those Sunday colour supplements should ask me to do a 'Day in the Life of . . .', it might sound something like this:

Neil Mackwood, born in 1950, is a journalist, writer and broadcaster who likes to eat, drink and attend parties. He has devoted the last few years of his life to high living, and has seen many of his colleagues fall by the wayside.

I wake up, like most successful people, very early in the morning. However, while they go to their offices, I go to the bathroom to get a glass of water because I feel dehydrated. I then return to bed and hope, dawn chorus willing, for a couple more hours of restless sleep before turning on the *Today* programme.

I then make my way to the kitchen where I brew myself a cup of tea – I can't face food. That swallowed, I lower myself into the hottest bath I can take, which makes me pink and sweaty – you can just smell the gin and tonic coming out – and afterwards climb into a suit. Whether it is crumpled depends on how it landed after being thrown off the night before. I then set off for Fleet Street on the tube, timing it so that I can be sure of getting a seat between Notting Hill Gate and Chancery Lane. Between the tube and the office I pass 'Chubbies' – a Fleet Street sandwich bar – where I may be tempted to buy a cheese roll to eat with the cup of coffee that is always ready on my arrival. Reviving over this, I read the papers and make my lunch arrangements before getting on with some work.

Journalism is said to be a sedentary profession so I make a point of walking briskly to my lunch appointment. At the restaurant I try to drink moderately through the three-course meal – no more than a bottle of wine each and only one brandy afterwards. To entertain properly is essential for business. Feeling much better, I catch a cab back to work because time is running short and there is work to be done. Full of bonhomie I phone my wife to check all is well with her and then grab a typewriter to decant the information that I have gleaned at lunch. Work out of the way, I proceed with colleagues to the pub to dissect our work over a parting drink.

Back home I wind down with some Mozart before discussing what's to eat for supper and which bottle of wine to drink. Afterwards I watch television – probably an imported soap opera and the snooker – and flop exhausted into bed at about midnight. The baby wakes at three o'clock, and I take the chance to have a glass of water before falling back into a wonderful deep sleep. Then it's six o'clock again and the circle is more or less repeated.

In fact it is not quite as bad as that. I play the odd game of squash, I don't smoke and I take the stairs instead of the lift. But after Catherine's gentle hints, I take a few naked twirls in the mirror and decide, with chest out, tummy sucked in and chin up, that I am a mesomorph – the type with bodies that are muscular, strong and altogether rather sportive – but which tend to run to fat. On reflection, I have to admit that I could be on the chubby side.**❞**

Neil

Is he (are you) overweight?

In 1983 the Royal College of Physicians conducted a survey on obesity in the UK, which showed that half the 20-year-old population tended to be overweight. With increasing age, the figure rose dramatically. About 30 per cent of men were found to be substantially overweight by their mid-twenties and by the age of 65 the percentage had risen to 54.

How dangerous it is to be overweight is not certain; other risk factors such as high blood pressure, an unhealthy diet and smoking may play an equal or greater part. However, if your man is, overweight, there are generally agreed risks to his health, in particular from heart disease and a tendency to high blood pressure and diabetes. It is also generally agreed that, although a sensible diet is vital to health, exercise – vigorous exercise in particular – controls weight and reduces the risks.

There are no rules about precisely what a man of a given height should weigh. It depends on his body type. The weights given in the table here are those recommended by the Royal College of Physicians. Obesity is defined as a weight 20 per cent or more above the upper "acceptable" weight range limit for each height.

Weight table — MEN

Height without shoes m (ft.in)	Weight without clothes kg (lb)		
	Acceptable average	Acceptable range	Obese
1.58 (5.2)	55.8 (123)	51-64 (112-141)	77 (169)
1.60 (5.3)	57.6 (126)	52-65 (115-143)	78 (171)
1.62 (5.4)	58.6 (129)	53-66 (117-146)	79 (174)
1.64 (5.4½)	59.6 (131)	54-67 (119-148)	80 (176)
1.66 (5.5½)	60.6 (133)	55-69 (121-152)	83 (182)
1.68 (5.6)	61.7 (135)	56-71 (123-156)	85 (187)
1.70 (5.7)	63.5 (139)	58-73 (128-160)	88 (194)
1.72 (5.8)	65.0 (143)	59-74 (130-163)	89 (196)
1.74 (5.8½)	66.5 (146)	60-75 (132-165)	90 (198)
1.76 (5.9)	68.0 (150)	62-77 (136-170)	92 (202)
1.78 (5.10)	69.4 (153)	64-79 (141-174)	95 (209)
1.80 (5.11)	71.0 (156)	65-80 (143-176)	96 (211)
1.82 (6.0)	72.6 (159)	66-82 (145-180)	98 (216)
1.84 (6.0½)	74.2 (163)	67-84 (147-185)	101 (222)
1.86 (6.1)	75.8 (166)	69-86 (152-189)	103 (227)
1.88 (6.2)	77.6 (170)	71-88 (156-194)	106 (233)
1.90 (6.3)	79.3 (175)	73-90 (160-198)	108 (238)
1.92 (6.4)	81.0 (178)	75-93 (165-205)	112 (246)

Weight table — WOMEN

Height without shoes m (ft.in)	Weight without clothes kg (lb)		
	Acceptable average	Acceptable range	Obese
1.45 (4.9)	46.0 (101)	42-53 (92-116)	64 (141)
1.48 (4.10)	46.5 (102)	42-54 (92-119)	65 (143)
1.50 (4.11)	47.0 (103)	43-55 (94-121)	66 (145)
1.52 (5.0)	48.5 (105)	44-57 (97-125)	68 (149)
1.54 (5.1)	49.5 (109)	44-58 (97-127)	70 (154)
1.56 (5.1½)	50.4 (111)	45-58 (99-128)	70 (154)
1.58 (5.2)	51.3 (112)	46-59 (101-130)	71 (156)
1.60 (5.3)	52.6 (115)	48-61 (105-134)	73 (160)
1.62 (5.4)	54.0 (119)	49-62 (108-136)	74 (163)
1.64 (5.4½)	55.4 (122)	50-64 (110-141)	77 (169)
1.66 (5.5½)	56.8 (124)	51-65 (112-143)	78 (171)
1.68 (5.6)	58.1 (127)	52-66 (114-145)	79 (174)
1.70 (5.7)	60.0 (132)	53-67 (116-147)	80 (176)
1.72 (5.8)	61.3 (134)	55-69 (121-152)	83 (182)
1.74 (5.8½)	62.6 (137)	56-70 (123-154)	84 (185)
1.76 (5.9)	64.0 (141)	58-72 (127-158)	86 (189)
1.78 (5.10)	65.3 (143)	59-74 (130-163)	89 (196)

Your man's mind

Physical fitness is not just a matter of the body. Your man's mental and emotional state is as much a foundation of his health as a strong heart and a sound pair of lungs. So, in order to get him truly fit, you must ask yourself the obvious question: *why is he so unfit in the first place?* Could the answer be any of the following: that his life is too pressurised; that he never relaxes properly; that he drinks too much – if so, is this out of habit or because he really feels he needs to?; that he smokes to help himself cope with the demands of work; that he drinks several cups of coffee a day to pep himself up; that he eats excessively to quell tension?

If some of these are his "coping methods", then your man may be overloading his system.

Years of this kind of self-neglect coupled with periods of extreme pressure, imposed by work and family responsibility, will grind the susceptible man down.

Stress

Stress is the very essence of life and when we are on the right side of it both physical and mental responses are enhanced and performances improved. There is a challenge to life which may be taxing and difficult but ultimately satisfying. Overstress – the killer – is when the job becomes too much, thoughts become agitated and confused, every day becomes a nightmare of joyless striving coupled with worrying physical symptoms.

"What do you mean? Of course I'm not affected by stress."

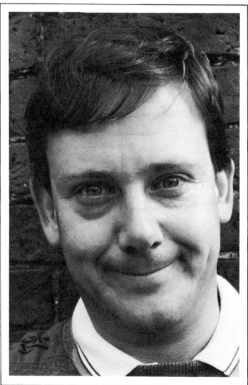 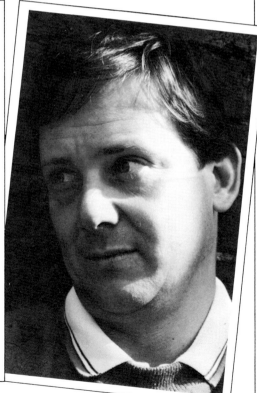

When the body does not get a chance to dissipate the chemical side-effects of stress by relaxation, rest or movement, the emotional and behavioural responses as well as the physical begin to suffer. Often a partner can see more clearly the subtle changes in behaviour patterns which are the warning signals of overstress. There is nothing like exercise and a good diet to keep your man operating efficiently and help him to keep things in perspective when the final tax demand comes through the letter-box, the house is discovered to be riddled with dry rot and he has been firmly routed in the office coup.

Every man has his own optimum performance level and particular tolerance of stress. Knowing how much pressure he can happily take is the best way to guard against breakdowns in health. Give him the stress self-assessment questionnaire to see in what ways stress affects him most and to give him an overall stress rating. Come back to it at monthly intervals during his shaping-up programme and compare the scores. You will be surprised by the improvement.

STRESS SELF-ASSESSMENT QUIZ

Score your answers:
Never *0*; Occasionally *1*;
Often *2*; Almost daily *3*.

During the last month, have you experienced these mental and emotional symptoms of stress?

1. Inability to concentrate
2. Difficulty in making simple decisions
3. Absent-mindedness
4. Loss of self-confidence
5. Irritability with others
6. Loss of interest in life
7. Extreme mood swings
8. Feelings of failure and inferiority
9. Uncalled-for aggression
10. Anxiety about imaginary misfortunes
11. Irrational fear or panic
12. Feeling helpless and unable to cope

During the last month, have you experienced these physical symptoms of stress?

1. Headaches
2. Difficulty in sleeping
3. Fatigue without exertion
4. Loss of appetite
5. Overeating binges
6. Indigestion
7. Constipation or diarrhoea
8. Nausea
9. High blood pressure
10. Colds or common flu
11. Skin rashes
12. Aching neck and shoulder muscles
13. Cramps and muscle spasms
14. Heart palpitations
15. Rapid breathing or breathlessness without exertion
16. Fainting spells
17. Sexual impotence
18. Fidgetiness or nervous mannerisms
19. Sweating without reason
20. Minor accidents

Add up your scores for your stress rating: 0-24 *low*; 25-48 *medium*; 49-72 *high*; 73-96 *very high*.

Talking him round

Don't be surprised if your suggestions about taking exercise, relaxing from work and cutting down on rich food, alcohol and cigarettes are met with such comments as: *"Fitness is fine for those who are lucky enough to have the time"; "This excessive self-interest currently in vogue seems extremely unhealthy to me";* or *"I don't know what you are worrying about. Winston Churchill lived to be 90 and he smoked, drank and ate every four hours – and took no exercise at all."*

In one sense he is correct: a puritanical life-style cannot guarantee health. The recent untimely death of the father of the jogging movement in the United States, Jim Fixx, gave ammunition to the anti-movement brigade (though his doctor had warned him not to run). Poor Mr Fixx – his number was up, 12 miles a day or not. But, although exercise will not necessarily increase the life-span, there is no doubt that the chances of a long life are dramatically influenced by a balanced way of living.

A long life

In 1982 Dr David Sobel, a pioneer in preventative medicine, in a talk entitled "Who Stays Healthy?", drew attention to research done in California on the life-styles of 7000 adults over a period of nine years. The results are striking. They found that, despite the progress of medicine, the very things that granny said were good for you were still the soundest basis for a long life. They were:

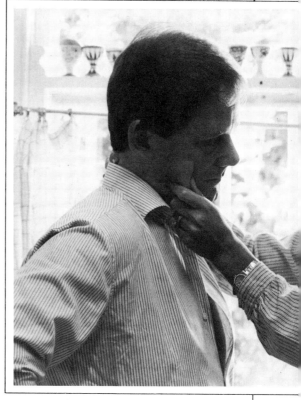

"I was but a spring lamb being coaxed gently to the slaughter." – *Neil*

> **1**
> **Get an average of seven to eight hours sleep a night.**
> **2**
> **Eat breakfast regularly.**
> **3**
> **Don't eat between meals.**
> **4**
> **Keep within a few pounds of your recommended weight.**
> **5**
> **Drink moderately or not at all.**
> **6**
> **Take regular physical exercise.**
> **7**
> **Don't smoke.**

Men aged 45 who had four or more of these good habits could expect to live 10 years longer than men who had only one of the habits. This does not mean that by serving your man breakfast regularly from now on you will ensure that he lives to be 85. Should you really wish him to be around for so long, then adequate rest and relaxation, sufficient but not excessive food and drink, and regular exercise will tip the balance in his favour.

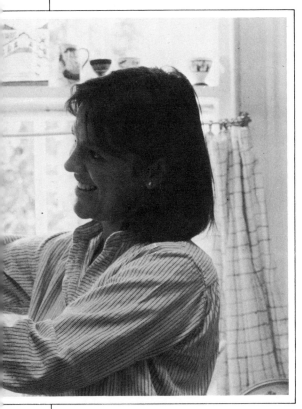

LIFE-EXPECTANCY QUIZ

The national average life-span for a man is 70 years (74 for women). Nobody can predict whether fate has floods, lightning, plague or runaway cars in store for you but it is possible to predict roughly what your chances of a long life are – and to improve considerably on those chances. There are always exceptions to every rule, but to get an idea of where you stand now do the following quiz.

	Score
Start with the number 70 (or 74 if a woman)	
Age	
If you are between 30 and 40	plus 2
If you are between 40 and 50	plus 3
If you are between 50 and 70	plus 4
If you are over 70	plus 5

Heredity	Score
If any of your grandparents lived to 85	plus 2
If all four grandparents lived to 80	plus 6
If either of your parents died of a stroke or heart attack before 50	minus 4
If a parent or sibling under 50 has/had a heart condition or diabetes since childhood	minus 3

Home environment	
If you live in a city of over two million people	minus 2
If you live in a village or town of under 10,000 people	plus 2
If you live with a spouse or friend	plus 3
But if you have long lived unhappily with a spouse or friend	minus 2
If you have lived alone since 25	minus 1 (for every 10 years)
But if you happily live alone	plus 2

Personal status	
If you have a degree or professional qualification	plus 2
If you earn over £40,000 a year	minus 2
If your income is under £4000 a year	minus 3
If you work behind a desk	minus 2
If your work requires regular physical activity	plus 2
If you are 65 or over and still working	plus 3
If you are happy	plus 1
If you are unhappy	minus 1

Life-style	
If you take vigorous exercise for at least 30 minutes four or more times a week	plus 4
If you take such exercise two or three times a week	plus 2
If you sleep more than 10 hours a night	minus 4
If you are aggressive and easily angered	minus 3
If you are easy-going and relaxed	plus 3
If you had a speeding charge in the past year	minus 1
If you smoke more than 40 cigarettes a day	minus 8
If 20 to 40 cigarettes	minus 6
If 10 to 20 cigarettes	minus 3
If you drink the equivalent of 1½oz of liquor a day	minus 1
If you are overweight by 50lb or more	minus 8
If by 30 to 50lb	minus 4
If by 10 to 30lb	minus 2
If you are over 40 and have annual checkups	plus 2

Total score gives your life expectancy

ffThe most ordinary days can throw up unusual situations which have dramatic consequences. I set off on a gentle joy-ride to Sussex to meet a friend of Catherine's. Little did I know that I was but a spring lamb being coaxed very gently to the slaughter. I knew something was amiss when an elegant man with a healthy complexion offset by a tan introduced himself as Dr Jan De Winter, and Catherine added that he was the Director of the Cancer Prevention Clinic in Brighton.

'Would you like a drink?'

'Yes, thank you.' (Of course I would.)

'Tea or coffee?'

'But this is gin and tonic time,' I thought. Then it dawned on me that the house was as dry as Ayer's Rock.

The sandwiches that followed provided another hint as to the philosophy of our temperance host. Surely this was not butter? – it wasn't. And surely this was wholemeal bread? – it was. And this was low fat, low cholesterol, low salt, low everything, chicken? – it was. The coffee was decaffeinated, the milk skimmed, the sugar bowl but a shelf ornament. I was getting the picture. Jan, charming as he was, was one of those doctors who don't smoke, don't drink, don't eat bacon and eggs, don't . . .

It was not long after we had exchanged a few pleasantries that he turned his attention to the life-style of the person sitting opposite him who was drinking his decaffeinated coffee and eating his wholemeal sandwiches. The spider had caught a victim.

'Why do you drink?' If I loved my wife, was I not being wholly selfish in drinking myself to death? What were my favourite flowers? – because he would like to know what to put on my grave. Did I realise that my life insurance premiums were probably more expensive than his? As if this wasn't enough, the spider then moved in to devour the fly in his web . . . *'And frankly, Neil, you are a little* obese.' By this time I was marvelling at the ability of the man to deliver body-blow after body-blow while still managing to be charming, and I didn't fully hear the rest of his speech – about fatness being a major cause of premature death.

Jan De Winter knows how to make a man feel guilty. It is, I suspect, his life's mission. He readily tells friends and casual visitors alike that as a senior consultant at the Royal Sussex County Hospital, Brighton, he has seen 12,000 patients into an early grave. In fact he is more precise and trots out the chilling figure of 12,327 which somehow brings home the terrible mortality rate. He has seen enough unnecessary death.

It was time to fight back and I mentioned the longevity of several hardened boozers I have known. *'Sheer luck,'* said Jan. My gloom was complete.

Several days after this depressing visit a book arrived through the post from Dr De Winter called *How To Die Young At Ninety*. It was full of such interesting titbits as: *'Five sugared cups of tea a day if taken for 50 years will have stimulated the pancreas 91,000 times'*, and it was inscribed *'To Catherine. A health guide whose simple message, when heeded, so lastingly affects our lives for the good. From Jan with love.'* I had little doubt as to whom the message was directed.

The visit to Dr Jan's led me to some careful self-examination. I recalled a party during which I heard someone remark, *'God, that man looks ill.'* On swivelling around, I realised to my chagrin that the subject of the remark was myself. Reflections in shop windows also confirmed that what the doctor had said about me was approaching the truth. I now entered a self-conscious stage when the bags under my eyes put Michael Aspel's in the shade. They were no longer characterful. Nor was my shape cuddly any more and I could not kid myself that certain discerning women, my wife included, found the not so gentle bulge around my waist an attractive and acceptable feature. All this, together with the realisation that not since school had I actually taken regular exercise, combined to make me want to tackle the problem.

The doctor had made a telling point about how the body – or perhaps more accurately the mind – is usually kind enough not to remind us of how sprightly we used to feel as teenagers. The process of deterioration happens too slowly to be noticed or cause concern. Sure, you can't touch your toes as easily as you once could or play five sets of tennis, or run up stairs two at a time without gasping for breath on every landing. But who wants to leap up stairs like a gazelle? And touching your toes is an unoriginal party piece. The downward path is a gradual one and you are lucky if you see a sign saying, *'Danger – engage a lower gear'*.

Now, late in the day, I saw the sign and decided to heed it, provided that my hugely enjoyable life-style would not be seriously affected. It was time for a de-coke. Like an alcoholic joining AA who first has to admit that he *is* an alcoholic, I had to admit to myself that there was a healthier way ahead that may, no must, be enjoyable. I did need help. **"**

Neil

Points of persuasion

The arguments are on your side, and though he might not be willing to admit it, he himself probably has a niggling suspicion that he could be fitter. Capitalise on these doubts. Use these points of persuasion:

☐*Overweight people run a very much higher risk of heart attacks and strokes, as well as of high blood pressure, diabetes, gall-bladder disease and arthritis. A sensible diet will reduce weight but exercise helps control obesity and does more to keep the body youthful.*

☐You are more susceptible to coronary heart disease, high blood pressure, diabetes, gall-bladder disease and obesity if members of your immediate family suffered from them. Controlling your weight and balancing your life-style reduce the risks.

☐*Exercise helps keep your blood pressure down. The "Tecumseh Project" studied 1700 men and found that the more active the men, regardless of age, the lower their blood pressure.*

☐The common disease of older people, atherosclerosis or arteriosclerosis, the hardening of the arteries – due to a build-up of fatty deposits including cholesterol – impedes the blood flow and can cause heart attacks or strokes. Exercise and sensible diet reduce risks.

☐*Repetitive exercise has been found to have the same calming effect on the mind as deep relaxation and meditation: the rhythm of the exercise and the concentration involved liberate people from day-to-day worries. If you find it hard to sit and contemplate or to lie down and relax, exercise is another way of settling the emotions.*

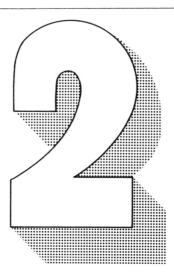

The Pleasure Principle

EXERCISE SHOULD BE PLEASURABLE. It should not hurt – whatever some fashionable pedlars of exercise programmes may say – and it should not be an onerous duty for which time has somehow to be found. A programme that can only be fulfilled by a few people willing to devote their lives to looking great is not what this book is about. Our three-month plan is based firmly on *the pleasure principle* and it can be realised even by men who have not thought of lifting a weight, swimming a stroke or jogging round the block in their lives. The three basic rules for success are:

1
The exercise must be enjoyable.
2
The programme must fit easily into daily life.
3
The inevitable discipline must not become a burden.

The pleasure principle means that you do what you want to do when you want to do it. This is not to say that missing out days from the programme will not have an effect. The only

sure way to shape up is to exercise consistently and the plan requires doing vigorous exercise three times a week in order gradually to build up fitness. If a week or more goes by without the body being used, the muscle cells will shrink, so if, for example, you go out running three times every week for several weeks, then remain in-active for three weeks, your fitness level will drop and you will need to build it up again.

The idea of the programme is not, however, for a man to fight himself into fitness but to ease himself into a more satisfactory way of living. There will inevitably be set-backs in achieving this if the programme is not followed consistent-ly but guilt should not be the driving force to continue. The motivation should come from the increasing feeling of well-being as your man gets fitter. Working on the pleasure principle, if he does not feel up to carrying out his planned exercise, perhaps because of a headache, over-work, a sleepless night, he should forget about doing it that day and not feel guilty about it.

Finding the time
If fitness becomes a battle between the time devoted to paying off the mortgage and the time

needed to take exercise, finally, after an initial burst of activity, the pursuit of the mortgage will win. But it is possible to make a plan even around the busiest of life-styles. One friend of ours takes his togs on his many business trips abroad and astonishes the locals by jogging in Baghdad. Another cycles to the City come heat-wave or blizzard and keeps deodorant and pin-stripes at work. A busy music impresario never misses his morning swim and has a taxi waiting outside the baths to whisk him to work after he has finished his twentieth length. An engineer who is confined to oil rigs for months on end takes with him his digital skipping-rope and notches up the numbers while counting the days before seeing land again.

Plan to set aside time that is not going to disrupt the daily routine. Early morning may be easier than the evening, or it may be possible to use lunch-times. A combination of times could be the best solution. Make the plan practical, part of an accepted weekly schedule, and exercise will soon become a pleasurable habit.

Personality

For some men, stacking an exercise routine on top of an already busy life may have counter-productive results. A workaholic, for example, may well adopt his exercise session in the same way that he runs his business life – striving for perfection, pushing on when tired, making his workout another of life's challenges – so that the time and effort invested bring poor dividends.

Dr Dorothy Harris of Pennsylvania State University, an authority on sports psychology, thinks that an aggressive, competitive approach to exercise is nevertheless better than taking no exercise at all. (Fine, if he doesn't happen to have high blood pressure.) She further contends that competitive exercise is a good way of monitoring how you cope with acute stress in the world outside the squash court, race-track or swimming bath. *"Action absorbs anxiety. Motion without emotion is useless, yet emotion without motion may be detrimental to health,"* she says. *"We think with our muscles. You don't just worry between your ears but with your whole body."*

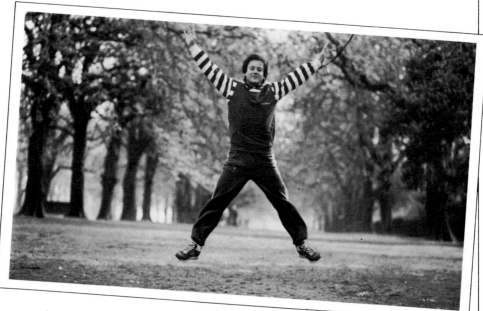

"I'm told that I should enjoy it regardless."

Research has been done by Dr David Glass of New York State University into personality types and the physical effects of competitive exercise. He used volunteers from a group that included what are termed A- and B-type personalities. Although everyone is likely to have characteristics of both types, A personalities tend to be aggressive and ambitious in business and sports, constantly preoccupied with meeting deadlines, impatient, punctual, quick speakers and eaters; B personalities, on the other hand, tend to be easy-going, uncompetitive and not overtly aggressive, contemplative, patient and unhurried.

Men of these different personalities were asked to take part in a game called 'superpong', each of them playing against a man who, unbeknownst to them, was a virtually unbeatable champion player from the research team. The first half of the game was played in silence but in the second half the champion player made such remarks as *"Can't you keep your eyes on the ball?"* or *"Christ, you are not even trying!"*. The effect of these insults on the A-type personalities was dramatic. Heart rate, blood pressure and adrenalin levels shot up whenever the remarks were made. They maximised the stress response, which is associated with coronary heart disease – a risk that the behaviour and life-styles of A-type personalities make greater.

❝It was important, so I was told, to know something about myself for this three-month regime. Odd, I thought. Never had I had to ponder on my psyche before playing cricket or competing in the 100-yard dash at school. We just went out and did it, though I remember my batting performances were badly affected by butterflies in the stomach – which became bats as I walked nearer the crease.

But times have moved on. Now, every national team in the world that actually wants to win something has its sports psychologist in the party. It's his job, roughly speaking, to ensure that on the day of competition the athletes achieve the potential that they reached in training. An athlete susceptible to pressure will feel, and in some cases be, physically sick with tension and, if he is to give of his best when it matters, all the stresses of competition must be removed from him.

What, you may ask, has this to do with me and my puny efforts to get fit? Only that it was impressed on me that I was not to enter the exercise programme in too competitive a frame of mind. I was to *enjoy* it! And to do this, I needed to be aware of my personality.

At about this time, I had one of those informal job interviews over a drink; and during this my attractive female interrogator asked me to define my personality. Cornered, I fell back on platitudes and half-truths. To say that I was hard-working, ambitious, aggressive when necessary, competitive and enthusiastic gave a good pointer to what I, the anxious applicant, felt were the qualities needed for the job. Whether the description conveyed much about my real character was another matter.

Afterwards, I began to think seriously about the question. Was I really aggressive, competitive, ambitious and hard-working? Was I not, rather, laid back, compliant, gregarious – too much so to reveal these characteristics at an interview if I did not want to be shown the door? OK, perhaps an element of my character is aggressive and impatient – my wife, family, friends, assure me that this is so – but I would not subscribe to the view that I am an archetypal A personality. True, I rave in traffic jams, chew at my fingers and curse the planners, but I do not believe that I am in fact the best driver on the

Sports specialist Dr Peter Sperryn points out the harm that may be done by not taking the right attitude to getting fit. The sedentary man who becomes a weekend exercise warrior with a Spartan belief that no exercise is good unless it gives him pain and pushes him beyond his limits may be putting himself at particular risk. As Dr Sperryn says, *"If we can't come to our sports and recreations as joyous pursuits, we may be better off not coming to them at all."*

Our programme to shape up will only be truly beneficial if it succeeds in dissipating some of the hassles and frustrations of life. If your man is aware of his personality type and how it may affect his approach to exercise, and to life generally, he is much more likely to achieve the well-being that is the overall aim. Getting your man to exercise in as non-competitive a way as possible is part of getting him properly fit.

Competition does not need to be ruled out entirely. If you suggest to a man with a wound-up, fiercely impatient personality that he sit down and learn deep-breathing techniques, he is not going to listen or, if he does take up the suggestion, he will probably become frustrated very quickly. Such a man may need some element of conflict in the exercise that he takes up. What matters is that the exercise is within his capacity and he is not striving for unrealistic goals that are to the detriment of his health.

---

road. True, I think it a waste of time to queue for 10 minutes at a sandwich bar – particularly when the end-product is so disappointing. True, I like to arrive at appointments, social and business, on time, and I like to think that if a thing is worth doing, it is worth doing properly.

Dr Dorothy Harris at least seems to be on my side in realising that men like me need to blow off a bit of steam now and then. This can be done with great effect in traffic jams – in winter anyway when the car windows are up; in Japan the frustrated motorist is even inclined to leap out of his car in a traffic jam to do strange exercises on the bonnet. Some behavioural therapist has in fact come up with a theory that swearing is good for you – it keeps down the blood pressure. However, my more usual habitat for the release of energy is not a traffic jam but a squash court, where a half-hearted effort guarantees that you come out the loser.

I have now, however, been told that if feelings of aggression are the driving force and they continue after the game, the benefits of the exercise and subsequent relaxation may be cancelled out. Aiming to win at all costs is evidently termed end-gaining – which I had previously thought was a Beckett play – and it is self-defeating. The overriding desire to win, win, win, only puts pressure on yourself and forces you to make mistakes. I have to tell myself that I should enjoy the game regardless of the result, although if I play so badly that I do not give my partner a worthwhile game, I can hardly be expected to whistle down the streets afterwards. To compete, and win, are important to me.

I recognised, however, that I had to be less competitive in my approach if the exercise programme was to work. Yes, a modicum of discipline was required but it did not matter if I missed a day or two out of the programme. I did not need to feel guilt; in these frenetic times I should be kind to myself. **"**

Neil

❝My object was to choose an exercise that would, as near as possible, be over very quickly, be painless, even fun, and would enable me to continue my life-style, though in modified form. I considered the alternatives.

Swimming was out. To me, it conjured up visions of verruca-infested pools, widdling infants, dive-bombing children and stinging eyes from chlorine-loaded water. More to the point, I swim like a crab and a good deal slower. I would be in there for hours.

Cycling was also a non-starter. I have no bike and have not been on one since school. I would probably have forgotten the art of keeping my balance. Besides, the idea of cycling in London struck me as far too dangerous. I'd be breathing in all the traffic fumes and getting stressed attempting not to end up underneath the 39 bus.

That left walking and jogging/running. Walking, however fast, was too slow for me, something to take up in my dotage. If I was going to be on my feet, I might as well run and be done with it. I couldn't claim to have ever shown any particular aptitude for running at school, which had the advantage that I was not likely to want to be competitive about it now. I imagined a nice 20-minute run in the morning, which wouldn't interfere with the rest of the day's work and pleasure. I'd choose a pretty course with flowers and trees to look at and would bid 'good morning' with a cheery wave to the people I passed. Afterwards I would cool down in the kitchen, sipping a cup of tea and imagining the weight that was streaming off. I would take it all nice and easy.

A few weeks ago it had seemed impossible that I would decide to join the ranks of joggers in the park with their absurd uniform of bandannas, leg-warmers, satin togs and personal stereos. But now I was in accepting mood, I would try to be positive. Would it, though, be possible actually to have fun doing this kind of thing?❞

Neil

Making the right choice of exercise

Choosing a form of exercise that suits the individual man is crucial to the success of the programme. The suggested alternatives given in the following chart are all forms of aerobic exercise. Aerobic means "with air" and it is used to describe vigorous exercise that is sustained for more than a brief period. The aim is to increase the amount of oxygen that a person can take up in relation to his or her body weight. The fitter the person, the more the oxygen capacity. The California-inspired aerobics craze has meant that aerobics is often associated with frenetic exercise classes to the sound of loud rock music and the aggressive shouts of an instructor about going for the burn. In fact aerobic exercise is comparatively gentle. Approached in the right way, it remains the quickest and most efficient way of improving your fitness level.

Any of the types of aerobic exercise suggested will produce fitness if carried out regularly according to the programme, but some have particular benefits and some suit particular body types. Consult the chart to work out the best choice. Above all, remember the pleasure principle: if the type of exercise does not appeal, the shaping-up programme is very likely to fail. Remember too that it is not necessary to choose only one form of exercise. He could, for example, jog on Monday, go for a swim on Wednesday and cycle to work on Friday.

Which exercise to choose

Type of exercise	Stamina/ endurance	Muscle strength	Relative benefits Flexibility of joints/suppleness of muscles	Trimness	Suitability
Walking	moderate to high provided undertaken energetically	low overall but quite high for leg muscles, especially calves	low except for hip joints in one range	helps hips and thighs; 150lb man uses c.230 cals per hour	all body types but especially endomorphs; recommended if very unfit, elderly or convalescent
Jogging/ running	high to very high, especially if running	high for leg muscles, especially calves	low except for hip joints in one range	helps hips and thighs; 150lb man uses c.600 cals per hour jogging, c.700 running	mesomorphs and ectomorphs in particular; not recommended if very overweight
Cycling	high if undertaken energetically	high for legs and back	high for knee and ankle joints; low otherwise	helps waist, hips and thighs; 150lb man uses c.600 cals per hour	all body types but especially mesomorphs and ectomorphs; recommended for the moderately overweight
Swimming	high if undertaken energetically	high for chest, back, shoulders, arms, legs	helps shoulder, hip and ankle joints; helps suppleness	helps waist and legs; 150lb man uses c.450 cals per hour	all body types but especially endomorphs; recommended if very overweight or back weak

Before you start

Before going any further, there are a few simple questions to be answered. It is important to answer the medical questionnaire first of all. The not too painful life-style test that follows will help your man find out how he rates on a healthy living scale. Afterwards come physical fitness tests to determine at what level – beginners, intermediate or advanced – he can start the 12-week course. This also gives him a point of comparison as he nurses his system back to health through the programme.

If any of the answers to the Medical Questionnaire are Yes, consult a doctor before undertaking any physical activity.

MEDICAL QUESTIONNAIRE

1. Has a doctor ever said that your blood pressure was too high?
2. Have you ever experienced pains in the chest or suffered from angina or heart trouble?
3. Are you recovering from an illness?
4. Do you have diabetes?
5. Are you more than 20lb overweight?
6. Do you ever feel faint or have spells of dizziness?
7. Do you suffer from backache, arthritis or any other pain in the joints?
8. Do you have asthma or breathing difficulties?
9. Has your doctor ever indicated that there are physical reasons why you should not take vigorous exercise?

LIFE-STYLE TEST

1. How often do you walk briskly for at least 20 minutes at a time?

	score
Four times a week	4
Twice a week	3
Once a week	2
Occasionally	1
Never	0

2. Do you engage in physical activity of sufficient duration to make you breathe hard (and/or perspire) for at least 15 minutes?

Four times a week	4
Twice a week	3
Once a week	2
Occasionally	1
Never	0

3. How would you describe the physical activity level of your work?

High	4
Above average	3
Moderate	2
Slight	1
Virtually non-existent	0

4. How do you feel when you wake up in the morning?

Energetic and lively	4
Reasonably lively	3
Alright	2
Tired	1
Exhausted	0

5. In the opinion of your wife/lover are you:

Slim	4
Normal	3
Chubby	2
Fat	1
Obese	0

6. According to the weight table on page 11, are you:

Within your acceptable weight range	4
1 to 5lb overweight	3
6 to 10lb overweight	2
11 to 19lb overweight	1
20lb or more overweight	0

7. Do you smoke?

	score
Never	4
Less than 10 a day	3
10 to 20 a day	2
20 to 30 a day	1
Over 30 a day	0

8. How much alcohol do you drink a week?

None/almost none	4
1 drink (pint beer, glass wine, measure spirits) a day average	3
2 to 3 drinks a day	2
4 to 5 drinks a day	1
6 or more drinks a day	0

9. What do you eat for breakfast?

Muesli sweetened with dry fruit/fresh fruit/ wholemeal bread/low fat margarine/boiled or poached egg/one cup tea or coffee with skimmed milk and no sugar	4
Fruit juice/wholemeal bread/butter/one cup tea or coffee with full-fat milk and no sugar	3
Cereal with sugar and full-fat milk/non-wholemeal bread/butter/two or more cups tea or coffee with full-fat milk and sugar	2
Fry-up of bacon and eggs/non-wholemeal bread/ butter/two or more cups tea or coffee with full-fat milk and sugar	1
Nothing	0

10. Which type of lunch do you eat most frequently?

Salad bar/light meal without alcohol	4
Desk (sandwiches/salads/fresh fruit) without alcohol	3
Pub (sausages/pasties/hamburgers/beans/chips) with beer/spirits	2
Business (three-course full-scale restaurant meal) with wine and liqueurs	1
Alcohol only, or nothing	0

Add up your score and take it over to add to your scores on the Physical Fitness tests that follow on the next page and pages 28-30.

Have a medical and your blood pressure checked at least every two years.

PHYSICAL FITNESS TESTS

Stamina

Stand in front of a bench or solid box (or use the stairs). Step up and down from the bench, alternating your leading foot, i.e. step up with your right foot, bring your left foot up beside it, then step down with your right foot and bring your left foot down beside it; repeat the movement beginning with your left foot. Try to establish an even pace of about 24 steps up per minute, and continue for two minutes. Ask your partner to time you so that you can concentrate on the rhythm of the exercise.

Wait two minutes, then take your pulse (see illustration). Count your pulse for 10 seconds and multiply by 6.

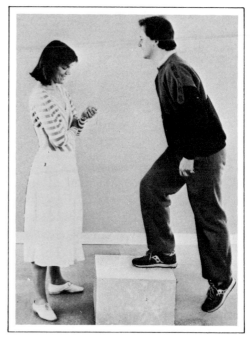

How many beats per minute?	score
75 to 90	4
90 to 105	3
105 to 120	2
120 to 135	1
135 plus	0

The Physical Fitness tests continue on page 28.

Taking your pulse

This can be done at either of the places shown below. Use your index and first finger to locate the pulse and begin timing when the second-hand of the watch reaches a point at which a 10-second interval can be easily distinguished.

If you count the carotid or neck pulse (left), never apply too much pressure with the fingers or you may cause the heart to slow, giving an inaccurate pulse count and possibly inducing faintness or dizziness.

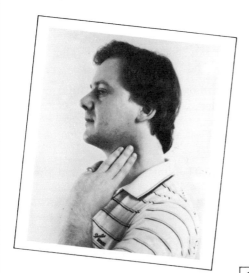

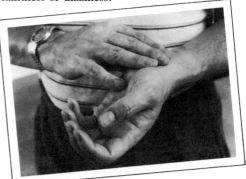

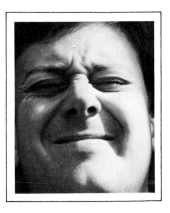

❝Honestly, you would think that I could run for nine minutes without stopping. That was to be the main part of the tests in the sports laboratory at Birmingham University, overseen by the eminent sports scientist Dr Craig Sharp. It was to be a day of awful reckoning.

I had made no special preparation for this test other than to dress in a tracksuit and wear a new, expensive pair of running shoes. The first thing they did was to remove half of the gear, leaving me shivering, white and near-naked in a pair of skimpy running shorts. Then, like a rat in a medical research lab, numerous leads were attached to various parts of my torso, presumably adjacent to vital internal organs. As if to silence any protest, a tube was placed in my mouth and – the final indignity – a plastic clothes-peg was attached to my nose. All these leads trailed off to a computer, which was to indicate to the staff if the trussed-up subject was about to have a seizure.

I was then coaxed on to a running platform, which soon hummed into action. I was instructed to run on it for nine minutes, at increasing speeds: first a warm-up 6mph, then 8mph, then 9mph. If at any time I felt as if I could not take it, I was to grab the handrails and lift my feet from the surface. However, I was sure that it was not too tall an order for one who played (irregular) squash and who could, if the occasion arose, run for a bus.

The first three minutes proved something of a shock to a system which, on reflection, had never been called on to run for a bus. I immediately began to regret the wine of the night before and spent the time considering the new regime – a gentle one, of course – that I was about to embark on. I would make a few concessions in order to help find the new me. For three months I would not taste beer, chocolates, hot cross buns, bacon and eggs, steak and chips, Cornish ice cream – and no more Stilton or tangy Cheddar, smelly Brie and French bread. This then was IT. What had I got myself into?

That took care of the first three minutes. I was breathing surprisingly hard and my wife was wearing one of her slightly concerned smiles. The increase of speed came as a jolt. Three miles an hour might not sound very much faster but the legs knew well enough that they were being asked to work harder. The heart too knew that this was no game of squash – "Where are the natural breaks?", it said.

Now, red of face and sweating, I began to realise that I might not get to the end of my allotted nine minutes – and what shame that would bring. The legs were turning to jelly, the heart was answering the pounding of my feet as the moving rubber road swept on and on. More and more I resembled a classroom hamster on a treadmill.

Somehow I kept going, only to hear a voice say 'Very good. Now be prepared for a change in speed ... to 9mph.' I had at least completed two-thirds of the allotted time –

but how was I going to manage the last three minutes? The smile on my wife's face had now turned to one of outright concern. My natural competitive spirit had determined that I would not humble myself in front of all these people by leaping off the treadmill, which was now whirring like a demented food-mixer, but it took all my resolve to stay on the machine. My legs seemed to be but a blur of incredible action, matched magnificently by my heart which had seen nothing like this. Amid this frenzy I was vaguely aware that a man of some authority – head of the department perhaps – had called in to see the phenomenon of an unfit man about to die in his lab. I could just hear him talking politely to the concerned wife above the din of the mad machine and the frequent clicks of the computer – now forecasting my imminent death.

'Two minutes to go,' said the instructor. By now I had used up all available energy and the process of putting one foot in front of the other was beyond my control. As the final horrible minute loomed, the whole apparatus came to a dramatic halt. Had I broken its will? Embarrassed apologies behind me indicated that the important-looking man who had entered the lab just before had inadvertently walked into an electric lead and brought the plug out of its socket. If I could, I would have bought him a pint.

A chair was provided for me and, still strapped to the wires and tubes, with nose-peg in place, I sat down to be monitored during an eight-minute recovery period. The fitter you are, the quicker the heart-beat returns to normal. Mine appeared to be so outraged at the pressure it had been placed under that it continued to beat as fast as a humming-bird's wing for the first few minutes. I did not feel well but at least I had a glow of satisfaction from thwarting the machine's design to break people down. Meanwhile, the computer chattered and the sweat poured.

Released from the tubes, showered and recovered (somewhat), I now faced a test that will-power alone could not help me pass – the dreaded 'pinch test'. A gruesome-looking pair of calipers was produced and applied to various fleshy parts of my body – the most revealing of all being just above the hip, where a roll of fat was quite evident however hard I tried to brace up. The calipers found what they were looking for – evidence of adipose tissue. In fact they found an estimated 22 per cent body fat, a statistic that enabled Dr Sharp to call me 'obese' without being intentionally rude.

So to the final test – one that reveals the shortcomings of smokers – to check the efficiency of the lungs. I took a vast breath and hurled it into a machine, which offered practically no resistance. I repeated this three times to achieve an average reading, and felt thoroughly faint.

In three months I will return to this sports laboratory with its cruel equipment and its clicking computers to find out if the plan has worked. My improvement, or lack of it, will be revealed. There can be no cheating.**"**

For the results of Neil's tests, see Dr Craig Sharp's report on page 92.

Body fat *right*

The pinch test is probably the easiest way to estimate the extent of excess body fat. Testing by submergence in a water tank is more accurate, but likely to pose practical problems, and for our purposes the pinch guideline will suffice. Make sure you are not maligning your man: excess body fat feels loose and soft whereas muscle is harder to the touch.

Have a ruler or tape-measure at hand. Pinch – gently – the flesh just above the hip and below the waist. Measure the distance along your thumb or forefinger.

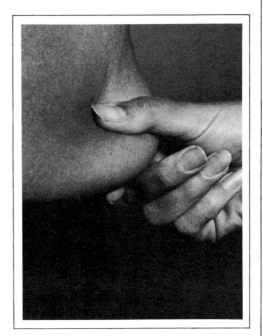

What is the measure?	score
½ inch or less	4
½ to 1 inch	3
1 to 2 inches	2
2 to 3 inches	1
3 inches plus	0

Suppleness *below*

Sit on the floor with your legs together, feet flexed (i.e. at right angles to leg). Keeping your back as straight as possible and stomach muscles pulled in, reach forwards with your hands and see if you can touch your feet.

How far are you able to reach?	score
Past your toes	4
To your toes	3
To your ankles	2
To mid calves	1
To knees	0

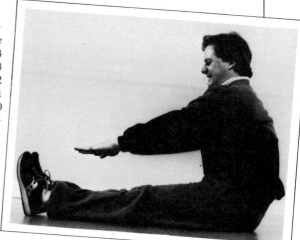

Muscular strength *below*

Lie on your back with your knees bent and your feet flat on the floor slightly apart, arms by your side. Breathe in. As you breathe out, push your lower back into the floor, pull your stomach muscles in strongly and curl your head and shoulders forwards, reaching for your knees with your hands, arms outstretched. See if you can touch your knees and hold the position for a count of 4. Then see if you can do the same exercise starting with your hands clasped behind your head and bringing your elbows to touch your knees?

How far can you reach?	score
Able to touch knees with elbows, hands clasped behind head, and hold for a count of 4	4
Able to touch knees with hands and hold for a count of 4	3
Able to touch knees with hands but not hold position	2
Able to reach forwards but not touch knees	1
Unable to raise body from floor	0

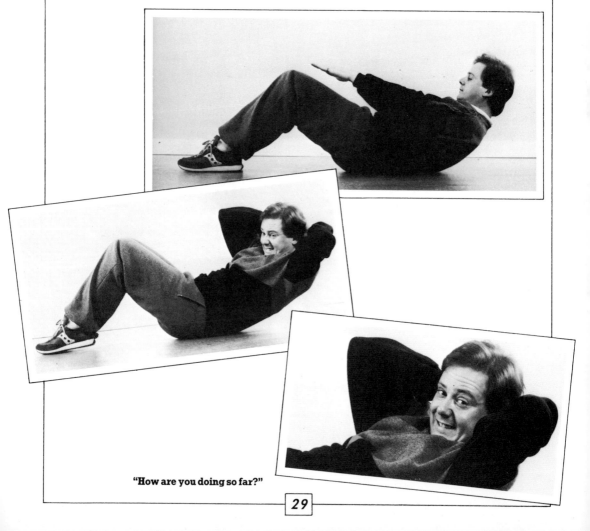

"How are you doing so far?"

Balance
Ask your partner to time you for this test. Stand
on one leg, foot flat on the floor, and bend your
other leg up behind you. Stretch your arms out
at shoulder height, then close your eyes.

How long can you last?	score
60 seconds or more	4
30 to 60 seconds	3
15 to 30 seconds	2
5 to 15 seconds	1
less than 5 seconds	0

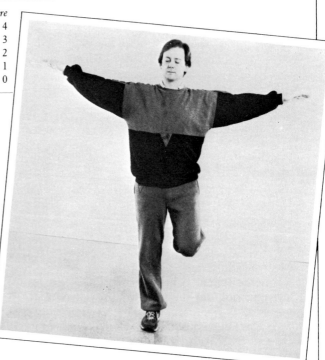

Now add up your scores from both the Life-style
and Physical Fitness Tests to find out which
12-week programme is most suitable for you.

Total score	Recommended programme
46 to 60	Advanced
31 to 45	Intermediate
30 and below	Beginners

❝Before I began my running, and still in my unredeemed state, I submitted to another set of tests, this time in a pleasant suburban villa in the west of London, home of chartered physiotherapist Vivian Grisogono. She is a healer of aches, injuries and pains, though the curious instruments of her trade would seem better placed in the basement of Madame Tussaud's. Soon I was to be made to climb upon something called a 'Masolet' machine, presumably designed for masochists, for the purposes of testing my 'dorsal rises', which until now I had innocently thought were something to do with trout fishing.

The tests were to evaluate my strength, co-ordination and flexibility. There would be just over a dozen exercises, each timed against a stop-watch, invigilated by Ms Grisogono and watched by Catherine. In three months I would return to be re-tested under similar circumstances to see if the programme had increased my all-round fitness.

Ms Grisogono is a no-nonsense type of person who might well be suited to an army job – regimental drill sergeant-major perhaps. You know the sort: indicate that you can do six press-ups and she's not happy until you have done nine and all the strength has ebbed away. The exercises that she had me doing were what used to be called 'gym' – and ever since I was made to hang on the wall bars for speaking out of turn at school, I have loathed 'gym'. Call the exercises strength and co-ordination tests if you like, but a 'squat' is a 'squat' – unless of course you are far from modern plumbing in Greece.

I remember in particular the 'calf toe-up' test, which was a lamb-in-leopard-skin sort of exercise. It sounded innocent enough – balance on one leg and rise on the toes – but taking the full weight of the body on one leg in this position turned out to be painful on the calf muscle. Cramp was never very far away. Then there was the 'hip abduction' test, which in itself sounds like a crime. It involved lying on my side, balanced upon my elbow and foot, and lifting my whole body up with a great grunt. And so on. The final test in the series was a simple matter of emulating a stork on one foot, closing the eyes and seeing how long it was possible to remain standing. I thought that I could last until next Sunday in this pose but I only managed 30 and 23 seconds on my right and left leg respectively. That meant I was not very body-aware; moreover I was utterly exhausted.

The idea was to test me to the full – so that every ounce of energy was extracted. This was made possible by the gently disparaging remarks that came my way from the sergeant with the stop-watch. I figured that if my body was about to break, I was surely in the right place to be put back together again, like Humpty Dumpty – who, I admit, I then passingly resembled.

When I returned three months later, the results, as the report on pages 94-5 shows, revealed a dramatic improvement. On the last test, for example, I managed to keep up the idiotic stork position for over two minutes on each leg – and only toppled over because I was getting bored. This proved conclusively that our exercise programme had reached all the parts that other exercise programmes do not reach.**❞**

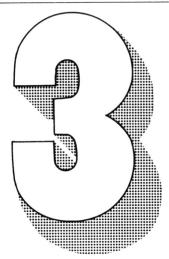

Going into Action

THE TIME HAS COME to put the 12-week exercise plan into action. The previous tests will have shown how fit – or unfit – your man is, and whether he should approach the programme as a beginner, or on an intermediate or advanced level. Whatever the level, the basic programme is the same. Its ingredients are summarised in the box on the right.

Try to spread the programme through the week as evenly as possible, although it can be varied to suit individual needs. Neil decided, for example, that he wanted his two days of rest to follow one another on Saturday and Sunday, leaving his weekends free. Occasionally, he broke this pattern because it proved impractical. A typical weekly timetable might look like this:

Day 1	**Aerobic exercise. Daily stretch.**
Day 2	**Rest. Daily stretch.**
Day 3	**Aerobic exercise. Daily stretch.**
Day 4	**Strengthening exercises. Daily stretch.**
Day 5	**Aerobic exercise. Daily stretch.**
Day 6	**Rest. Daily stretch.**
Day 7	**Strengthening exercises. Daily stretch.**

THE WEEKLY PROGRAMME INGREDIENTS

Aerobic exercise
walking, jogging/running, cycling, swimming – three times a week for between 10 and 60 minutes according to the level. This is preceded by a 5- to 15-minute warm-up, consisting of mobilising exercises, pulse-warmers and stretch exercises, and finishes with a short cool-down period.

Stretch exercises
using the same exercises as in the warm-up, every day for 5 to 10 minutes, plus optional stress-reducing stretches to be done whenever needed.

Strengthening exercises
twice a week for 10 to 20 minutes. These are graded on three levels, with optional additional exercises working with weights.

Rest
twice a week.

Aerobic Exercise

How much exercise you can take varies greatly from person to person and from time to time. Everybody has a different capacity, depending on age, sex, weight, current state of fitness and hereditary factors. These determine the efficiency of your heart and circulation, together with the efficiency of oxygen extraction in the muscles. Aerobic exercise dramatically improves that efficiency by training the body to work harder, but the training must be within a person's capacity if it is to be effective.

Finding the "Training Zone"

To ensure that you are exercising within your capacity – or, to use sports terminology, within your training zone – you need to measure your heart rate. Whether you exercise on a beginners, intermediate or advanced level, your aim should be to work the heart at 70 to 85 per cent of its maximum rate, for a minimum period of 10 minutes. If you are doing this, you are within your training zone and will get most benefit from exercising. If you work below it, you will not improve your fitness level; above it and you will be at risk of straining yourself.

The maximum heart rate can be calculated approximately by subtracting a person's age from 220; 70 to 85 per cent of the resulting figure gives the training zone (*see table below*). Note, however, that the rates given are averages only. A third of the population may have a higher or lower maximum heart rate for age, and the training zone figures would differ accordingly.

Heart rates and the Training Zone

Age	MHR*	70%/85% MHR*	Age	MHR*	70%/85% MHR*	Age	MHR*	70%/85% MHR*
20	200	140	170	41	179	125	152	62	158	110	134
21	199	139	169	42	178	125	151	63	157	110	133
22	198	139	168	43	177	124	150	64	156	109	133
23	197	138	167	44	176	123	150	65	155	108	132
24	196	137	167	45	175	123	149	66	154	108	131
25	195	137	166	46	174	122	148	67	153	107	130
26	194	136	165	47	173	121	147	68	152	106	129
27	193	135	164	48	172	120	146	69	151	106	128
28	192	134	163	49	171	120	145	70	150	105	128
29	191	134	162	50	170	119	144	71	149	104	127
30	190	133	161	51	169	118	144	72	148	104	126
31	189	132	161	52	168	118	143	73	147	103	125
32	188	132	160	53	167	117	142	74	146	102	124
33	187	131	159	54	166	116	141	75	145	101	123
34	186	130	158	55	165	116	140	76	144	100	122
35	185	130	157	56	164	115	139	77	143	100	122
36	184	129	156	57	163	114	138	78	142	99	121
37	183	128	155	58	162	113	138	79	141	99	120
38	182	127	155	59	161	113	137	80	140	98	119
39	181	127	154	60	160	112	136				
40	180	126	153	61	159	111	135				

MHR = Maximum Heart Rate

Taking Your Pulse

Because it is important to know whether you are exercising within your training zone, you should take your pulse – a measure of your heart rate – before, during and after strenuous exercise. After a while, you will become aware instinctively whether you are working within your target and will not need to check your heart rate. However, in the early stages in particular, check your pulse before exercising, 5 minutes into the warm-up and 5 minutes into the cool-down. How to take your pulse is shown on page 25.

If you have had a heavy night out or a hard day at the office, you may find that your pulse is up from its normal "resting rate" by about 10 beats. Whenever that is the case, exercise more slowly or delay your exercise until the next day.

The Warm-Up

The purpose of the warm-up is to prepare the heart and lungs, and the muscles and joints, for the extra work that they are about to take on. It consists of three parts: mobilising exercises, primarily to ease the joints into work; pulse-warmers to ready the heart and lungs; and stretch exercises for the muscles, which vary slightly according to which form of aerobic exercise you intend to do. The time taken is small – 5 to 15 minutes – but the warm-up should never be missed because:

Sudden, heavy strain on the heart and lungs is avoided. Such strain can be damaging and even fatal for an extremely unfit person.

Aches and pains in the joints are much less likely. The mobilising exercises allow the cartilages to absorb fluid that acts as a protective cushion around the joints.

The risk of cramp and muscle tears or stiffness is considerably reduced by the improvement in circulation as a result of stretch exercises.

Breathing is made more efficient by reducing the tightness in the chest, shoulders and ribcage.

Tension is released, which increases overall energy.

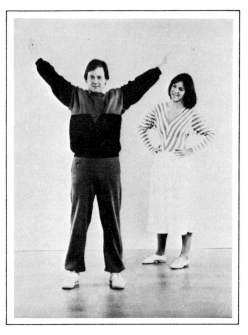

Mobilising Exercises

The five exercises here form the first part of the warm-up. Each exercise should be done for about 30 seconds in the short, 5-minute warm-up, and for one minute or more in the longer, 15-minute warm-up.

Pulse-warmers

This part of the warm-up consists of any exercise performed quickly, so that the heart and lungs are prepared for extra work. The exercise should be done for 30 seconds to one minute, followed by a rest period of 15 to 30 seconds. Beginners could repeat one of the mobilising exercises here or do one of the strengthening exercises on pages 49-54. Intermediate or advanced levels might choose to run on the spot, skip or do one of the strengthening exercises on pages 55-60 and 61-67.

WARM-UPS

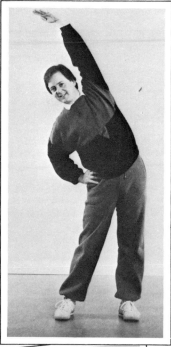

 1
FAR LEFT
Stand with feet apart. Circle arms backwards over your head and lower to your sides in one continuous movement. Try not to arch your back.

 2
LEFT
Stand with feet apart, one hand on your hip. Stretch the other arm over your head and bend to the side, stretching further. Repeat for about 15 seconds on each side.

 3
BELOW LEFT
Stand with feet apart, arms outstretched at shoulder height. Swing your arms to the right, looking over your right shoulder and clenching your bottom to hold your hips forward, then swing to your left. To be done in one continuous movement.

 4
BELOW CENTRE
Stand with feet apart, knees slightly bent, and circle your hips, swinging your weight over each leg.

 5
BELOW RIGHT
Stand with legs apart, feet turned outwards and hands on hips. Bend your knees, then straighten them, pulling up strongly above the knee. To be done in one continuous movement.

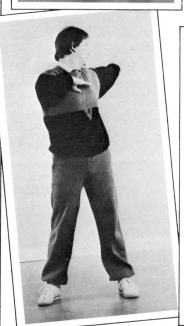

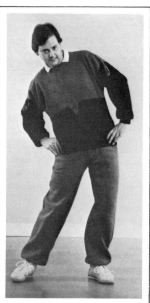

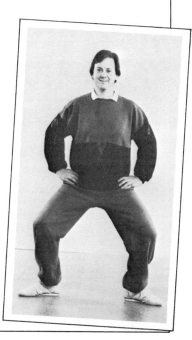

The Cool-Down

To cool down after strenuous exercise is as important as to warm up and for similar reasons. If the body comes to a sudden halt, the heart has to work very hard to prevent the increased blood supply to the legs pooling in the muscles and upsetting the general blood flow through the body. The brain may be left short of oxygen and you may feel dizzy and could even faint. Also, the waste products that are built up during exercise cannot be efficiently disposed of, which increases the chances of muscle stiffness.

The cool-down is simply a slowing down of activity after vigorous exercise in order to prevent such problems. If you have been exercising for 20 minutes or more, allow a recovery period of 5 to 8 minutes. If you have been running, for example, you might slow to a gentle jog and then to walking at decreasing speed before coming to a halt. It will become obvious how much time you need to cool down; as you become fitter, your body will adjust to normal more quickly.

Rest

Rest is an essential component of the programme, as long as rest days don't end up stretched into weeks! Give yourself two days complete break from vigorous exercise a week. Doing too much is as bad as doing too little – but remember that if you rest for too long, you will lose the benefits of your earlier work.

Safety Rules

There are bound to be times when you are not sure if it is safe for you to exercise. Always consult a doctor if you are in serious doubt, and stick to the following guidelines.

If exercise hurts, stop. There is a marked difference between working strongly and feeling pain. Always treat pain as a warning signal.

Do not exercise if you are ill. In most cases, the reason why people collapse on runs or playing squash is that they were already ill and not that they were overdoing it.

After a break from exercise for whatever reason – holidays, work, injury, illness – **do not start again at the level where you left off.** Begin at a lower level, or go back to the starting point, and gradually build up your fitness.

Do not exercise on a full stomach. When you exercise, the stomach stops digesting and if you have just had a meal, you will feel very uncomfortable and will be liable to strain yourself. Leave at least an hour after a big meal and half an hour after a light snack before exercising.

Always warm up before doing vigorous exercise and always allow for a cool-down period at the end.

Wear the correct clothing, which should allow free movement, and shoes that are comfortable and designed for exercise.

The Aerobic Programme

Whichever form of aerobic exercise has been chosen, it needs to be approached progressively. The charts on pages 39, 42 and 45 give the times or distances to be aimed for over the 12-week programme at beginners, intermediate or advanced level. These times or distances are guidelines only. They should not be taken as gospel or produce guilt if they are not met. Nor should they be taken as a challenge. There are no congratulations in store for breaking records, as Neil discovered.

At the beginners' level, the time taken up by exercise is as little as 10 to 20 minutes, excluding the essential few minutes to warm up and cool down, on three days of the week. Even at the advanced level, no more than an hour's sustained vigorous exercise is advised, although at this level the programme suggests including a fourth session in some weeks and a change to a more strenuous pace on some days. The benefit from doing more than the three sessions a week that are necessary to achieve fitness is small in return for the extra time and it is only when an advanced level of fitness has been reached that the small additional gain is worth considering. However, most people who are this fit want to do an extra session, not so much to get to the peak of fitness but for sheer enjoyment.

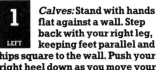

JOGGING WARM-UPS

WALKING

For many people, walking is the most convenient form of aerobic exercise to take. It requires no special clothing, no extras such as a bicycle to consider, and it can be done almost anywhere at any time. The elderly and the very unfit may find it particularly suitable and, if wished, they can progress from walking to gentle jogging and even running as their fitness improves. Walking must, however, be brisk and sustained if it is to have benefits.

Stretch Exercises for walking, jogging and running

Each of the following five exercises should be done for 10 to 30 seconds as part of your warm-up, and should be done separately for 30 seconds each as your daily stretch (see page 46).

TIPS FOR WALKING

- Wear a strong pair of good fitting shoes and comfortable clothes.

- Maintain a good posture; the looser the upper body, the better the walk.

- Make sure that the heel of the foot touches the ground firmly and push off strongly from each step with the back leg to use the buttocks as much as possible.

- Walk in pleasant surroundings and avoid difficult surfaces.

- As a beginner, allow for the extra effort required on hills and when facing winds.

- Walk with a friend whenever you can.

1 LEFT *Calves:* **Stand with hands flat against a wall. Step back with your right leg, keeping feet parallel and hips square to the wall. Push your right heel down as you move your hips forward. Hold. Repeat with your left leg.**

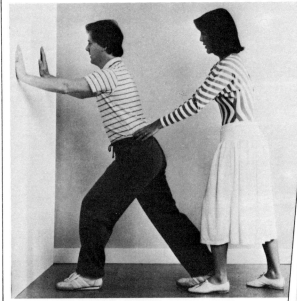

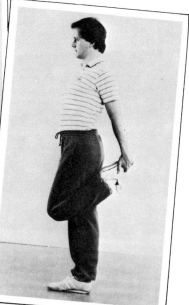

2 RIGHT *Thighs:* **Balance on one leg and bend your other leg up, holding on to your foot or ankle. Keep your hips well forward and gently pull your heel towards your bottom. Hold. Repeat with other leg.**

JOGGING and RUNNING

The dividing line between jogging and running is difficult to define. One is an extension of the other, and both are extensions of walking and have similar advantages of convenience provided that you are prepared to brave the English weather. Exercising by jogging or running fits easily into life; it can be done before or after work, at lunchtime in a nearby park, over the weekends, and alone or in company. It brings quick rewards – greatly improved stamina, weight control and overall well-being – which accounts for its popularity among people from all walks of life. If you are extremely unfit or overweight, it is advisable to begin with brisk walking and progress to jogging, or you may prefer to swim or cycle.

TIPS FOR JOGGING AND RUNNING

- Wear trainers with well-cushioned soles; for extra protection, replace the insoles with Sorbothane insoles.

- Wear light-weight clothing – synthetic fabrics are more convenient – and, if running at night, wear luminous arm bands. Avoid wearing tennis shorts, which do not allow for sufficient movement.

- Maintain a good posture, keeping the shoulders and arms relaxed.

- Make sure that the heels come down each time the foot hits the ground; this prevents a build-up of tension in the calves.

- Be aware of the rhythm of the run and change pace from time to time.

- Vary the running surfaces between roads, grass and cinder; the softer the surface, the more comfortable the run.

- Run in pleasant surroundings and vary the routes.

- Run with a friend when possible.

- Remember road safety and other people: face the on-coming traffic, look ahead at the road surface for possible pitfalls and allow for pedestrians on the path.

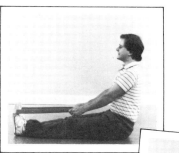

3 ABOVE *Backs of legs:* Sit on the floor, knees bent, and place a belt round the bottom of your feet. Keeping your back straight and pulling on the belt, stretch out your legs till the backs of your knees are straight. Hold.

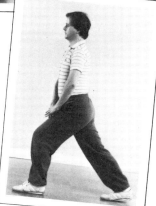

4 LEFT *Hips:* Stretch one leg out straight behind you and bend the other leg, resting your hands on the thigh. Your knee should be directly aligned over your ankle. Move your trunk downwards as far as you can, keeping your back leg straight. Hold.

JOGGING WARM-UPS

WALKING, JOGGING or RUNNING programme

Week 1 *minutes*	Beginners	Intermediate *miles*	Advanced *miles*	Week 7 *minutes*	Beginners	Intermediate *miles*	Advanced *miles*
day 1	10	2	5 steady	*day 1*	19	3	6 steady
day 2	10	2	3 fast	*day 2*	15	4	4 steady
day 3	10	3	4 steady	*day 3*	12	3½	4 steady
Week 2				Week 8			
day 1	12	2	5 steady	*day 1*	19	3	3 fast
day 2	10	3	2 fast	*day 2*	15	4	6 steady
day 3	12	3	4 steady	*day 3*	19	4	3 fast
(day 4)			2 fast	*(day 4)*			4 steady
Week 3				Week 9			
day 1	14	2	5 steady	*day 1*	21	3	5 steady
day 2	12	3	3 fast	*day 2*	19	4½	6 steady
day 3	14	3½	5 steady	*day 3*	15	4	5 steady
Week 4				Week 10			
day 1	14	2	3 fast	*day 1*	23	3	3 fast
day 2	12	4	5 steady	*day 2*	15	5	6 steady
day 3	14	3	2 fast	*day 3*	19	3	2 fast
(day 4)			5 steady	*(day 4)*			5 steady
Week 5				Week 11			
day 1	15	2	5 steady	*day 1*	23	4	6 steady
day 2	10	3	5 steady	*day 2*	19	5	5 steady
day 3	15	4	5 steady	*day 3*	19	3	6 steady
Week 6				Week 12			
day 1	17	3	4 steady	*day 1*	25	5	6 steady
day 2	15	3	6 steady	*day 2*	15	4	6 steady
day 3	10	4	3 fast	*day 3*	20	4	6 steady

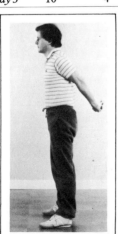

5 LEFT & RIGHT

Shoulders: Clasp your hands behind your back and turn the palms outwards. Standing straight, bring your arms up towards your head as far as they will go, keeping them straight. With your stomach held in, lean forwards, bending your knees and bringing your arms up as far as possible.

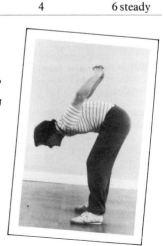

CYCLING

Cycling can be started at any level of fitness and has the advantage, particularly if you are overweight, that it does not tax the joints of the body. Like the other forms of aerobic exercise, it improves stamina provided that the effort put into it is consistent. Speed is not the object but to keep up a steady pace for a period of time (*see chart overleaf*).

If you are able to cycle to work, your shaping up programme will hardly conflict at all with your daily timetable. Part of the journey could be by train and part by bike – British Rail generally allows bicycles in guard's vans free of charge. Or you might use a collapsible bike so that you can drive to work or into the country and then cycle to appointments at lunchtime or other times during the day, or make cycling trips round the countryside.

TIPS FOR CYCLING

- Wear hard shoes rather than trainers, and use toe-clips and straps to improve balance.

- For more serious cycling or if you sweat a lot, wear a tracksuit; keep a change of clothes at work if necessary.

- Wear luminous arm bands or sashes, and ensure that you and the bike are visible (particularly essential at night).

- Check that the bike is the right size for you; when you stand astride the bike, your feet should be flat on the ground and the cross-bar just below your crotch.

- Balance your weight evenly between the handlebars, pedals and saddle to avoid aches and pains.

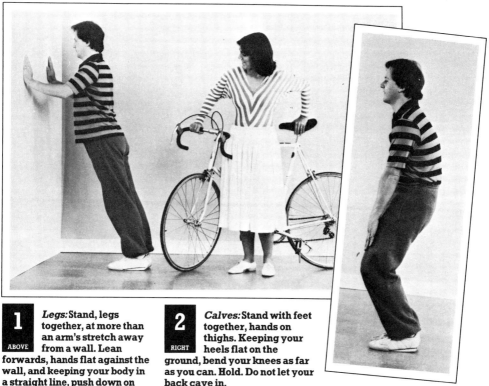

1 ABOVE **Legs:** Stand, legs together, at more than an arm's stretch away from a wall. Lean forwards, hands flat against the wall, and keeping your body in a straight line, push down on your heels. Hold.

2 RIGHT **Calves:** Stand with feet together, hands on thighs. Keeping your heels flat on the ground, bend your knees as far as you can. Hold. Do not let your back cave in.

Stretch Exercises for cycling

Each of these five exercises should be done for 10 to 30 seconds as part of your warm-up, and should be done separately for 30 seconds each as your daily stretch (see page 46).

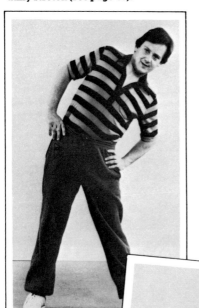

- Ride with the saddle tipped slightly upwards.
- If you get backache, try raising the handlebars or altering the saddle height.
- Stand up in the pedals when going uphill in order to avoid knee-cap pain (but note that this may require practice).
- Bend your arms when going over bumps to help cushion the impact.
- Keep the tyres well pumped for a smoother ride.
- Choose pleasant surroundings and cycle in company.

5 **BELOW** *Shoulders and sides of trunk:* **Stand with legs apart. Lift arms above your head and hold your right elbow with your left hand. Keeping stomach in, stretch to the left. Repeat on the right side.**

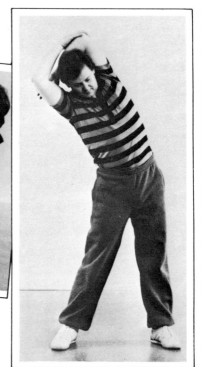

3 **ABOVE** *Inside legs and sides of trunk:* **Stand with legs wide apart, hands on hips. Keeping the back straight, lean to one side as far as you can and hold. Repeat, leaning to the other side.**

4 **ABOVE RIGHT** *Thighs and ankles:* **Kneel with legs slightly apart and feet running parallel to the sides of your bottom. Put hands behind you, push hips forward and lean back. (If your ankles are very tight, sit on a cushion.)**

CYCLING programme

	Beginners *in minutes*	Intermediate *in minutes*	Advanced *in minutes*		Beginners *in minutes*	Intermediate *in minutes*	Advanced *in minutes*
Week 1				Week 7			
day 1	15	35	50	*day 1*	20	40	60
day 2	15	35	50	*day 2*	25	45	60
day 3	15	35	50	*day 3*	25	40	50
Week 2				Week 8			
day 1	20	35	50	*day 1*	20	45	50
day 2	15	40	30 fast	*day 2*	30	40	30 fast
day 3	15	35	50	*day 3*	25	45	50
Week 3				*(day 4)*			40 fast
day 1	20	35	50	Week 9			
day 2	15	35	30 fast	*day 1*	25	40	60
day 3	20	40	40	*day 2*	30	45	40 fast
(day 4)			30 fast	*day 3*	30	45	50
Week 4				*(day 4)*			30 fast
day 1	20	35	50	Week 10			
day 2	20	40	40 fast	*day 1*	25	45	60
day 3	20	40	50	*day 2*	30	45	60
(day 4)			30 fast	*day 3*	35	45	60
Week 5				Week 11			
day 1	20	40	50	*day 1*	30	45	60
day 2	15	40	30 fast	*day 2*	30	50	40 fast
day 3	25	40	60	*day 3*	35	45	60
Week 6				*(day 4)*			40 fast
day 1	15	35	50	Week 12			
day 2	25	40	60	*day 1*	30	50	60
day 3	25	45	50	*day 2*	35	50	50 fast
				day 3	35	50	60

"Cycling as a choice of exercise was out. I have no bike and have not been on one since school. Besides the idea of cycling in London struck me as far too dangerous. I'd be breathing in all the traffic fumes and getting stressed attempting not to end up under the 39 bus."

– Neil

SWIMMING
WARM-UPS

SWIMMING

One of the greatest advantages of swimming is that the weight of the body is not a handicap. If you are carrying an extra couple of stone, exercising in water avoids putting your joints under strain, whereas jogging would carry this risk – apart from probably not being enjoyable. It is therefore worth thinking seriously about swimming if this is your problem, even if you have done little swimming before; once you have reduced your weight by a stone or more, you could swap to another form of aerobic exercise.

Swimming is extremely effective in improving the general tone of your body, which is the result of the muscles being worked against the resistance of the water. It is, however, more difficult to achieve the "aerobic effect" – the quick improvement to the cardiovascular system – by swimming than it is by jogging because only proficient swimmers can sustain the vigorous pace necessary.

Beginners should take it slowly, with rests between widths or lengths, and progress from backstroke to sidestroke, breaststroke and finally, for the fit, crawl. The stroke is less important than keeping up a steady pace over a period of time.

Stretch Exercises for swimming

Each of the following five exercises should be done for 10 to 30 seconds as part of your warm-up, and be done separately for 30 seconds each as your daily stretch (see page 46).

1 LEFT *Shoulders and arms:* Stand beside a wall, with your right leg forward and left leg stretched out straight behind you. Stretch your right arm back along the wall at shoulder height. Bend your right leg and tuck in your bottom. Pull back on your left shoulder as you move the right shoulder forwards. Repeat on left.

2 RIGHT *Shoulders and back:* Place your hands on a ledge or back of a chair. Bend your knees and try to flatten your back so that your arms and back are at right angles to the ledge. Let your head hang down.

3 BELOW

Shoulders, chest and back: Hold a swimming towel in front of you, hands about 9 inches apart. Round your back and push your hands away from you as hard as possible. Hold. Then straighten your back, widen your grip and lift your arms over your head, stretching out behind you. Hold.

TIPS FOR SWIMMING

- Wear goggles to protect your eyes from the effects of chlorine; use eye-drops if irritation is a problem.

- If you wear contact lenses, check that they are suitable for wearing in water: hard lenses tend to float off the eye.

- Avoid getting cold in the water, which may cause cramp.

- If your neck becomes tense when swimming breaststroke, you are very probably carrying your head too high in the water. Swim side-stroke or backstroke instead, and arrange for some coaching to counteract the problem.

- Avoid doing butterfly stroke if you have lower back problems.

- Swim crawl rather than breaststroke if you suffer from knee problems.

- Check with the pool staff when the quietest times are to see if you can take advantage of them; some baths have reserved sessions for adults and for men or women only.

- Swim with a friend if possible.

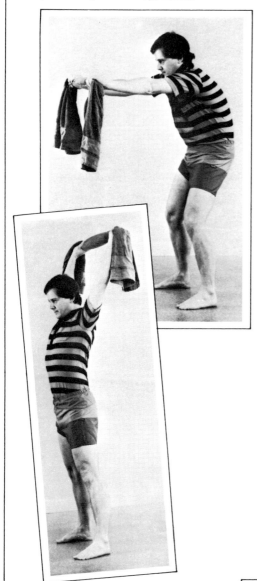

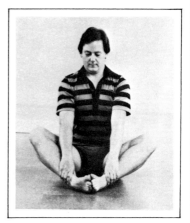

4 ABOVE

Hips and groin: Sit on the floor, soles of your feet together. Hold your ankles and straighten your back. Breathe in and as you breathe out, push your knees towards floor. If you can, lean forwards with straight back.

SWIMMING WARM-UPS

SWIMMING programme

Week 1	Beginners *in minutes*	Intermediate *in minutes*	Advanced *in minutes*
day 1	10	20	35
day 2	10	20	35
day 3	10	20	35
Week 2			
day 1	10	20	35
day 2	12	20	35
day 3	10	24	40
Week 3			
day 1	10	20	35
day 2	12	24	40
day 3	12	24	35
Week 4			
day 1	12	24	35
day 2	12	24	40
day 3	12	24	40
Week 5			
day 1	10	24	40
day 2	15	24	30 fast
day 3	12	28	40
Week 6			
day 1	12	24	40
day 2	15	28	40
day 3	12	28	30 fast

Week 7	Beginners *in minutes*	Intermediate *in minutes*	Advanced *in minutes*
day 1	12	28	30
day 2	15	15 fast	30 fast
day 3	15	20	30
(day 4)			30 fast
Week 8			
day 1	15	30	40
day 2	15	15 fast	30 fast
day 3	15	24	40
(day 4)			30 fast
Week 9			
day 1	15	30	40
day 2	18	30	40
day 3	15	18 fast	40
Week 10			
day 1	15	30	40
day 2	18	30	40
day 3	18	15 fast	45
Week 11			
day 1	18	35	40
day 2	18	30	35 fast
day 3	18	30	40
Week 12			
day 1	20	35	45
day 2	15	30	40
day 3	18	35	45

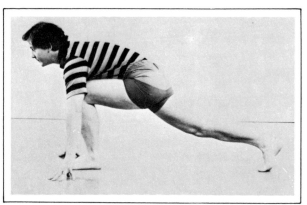

Beginners should swim any stroke; intermediate and advanced levels should vary their swimming strokes during each session.

5
LEFT

Hips: Kneel on all fours. Step forward with your right leg, keeping your knee aligned above your ankle. Stretch left leg straight out behind you. Hold. Repeat with other leg.

Stretch Exercises

A daily stretch increases overall flexibility and is an excellent way of keeping the body trim and supple. Use the stretch exercises for the warm-up, shown on pages 37-45, as a separate 5- to 10-minute routine every day. You can repeat the exercises for the particular type of aerobic exercise that you are doing, or you can use those for other types, varying them to suit yourself. Each stretch exercise concentrates on muscles in one area of the body so that you can work on, for example, your shoulders or legs if these are weak areas or if you want to increase the flexibility of these muscle groups.

Stretch away the stress

The body is shaped by the way that it is used – as the increasing girths of men with sedentary life-styles show only too well – but often it is not only the waistline that suffers. Headaches, neckaches and backaches are all familiar to the desk-bound and car-bound man, and woman. They are frequently the result of physical tension. Most of the movement in the body is created by muscle contraction and if the contraction is held for a long period, for example, if you remain hunched over a desk, tension develops.

As you progress through the 12-week course, problems connected with physical tension should gradually fade but there are always times when they will crop up. The following simple stretch exercises, devised by the Bodyworkshop, help reduce physical tension and can be done whenever the need arises.

1 LEFT **Clasp your hands round the top of your head towards the back, letting your elbows hang down loosely. Breathe in. As you breathe out, drop your chin and relax the shoulders. (You should feel a gentle pull down the back of the neck.) Hold the stretch, breathing normally, for 30 to 60 seconds.**

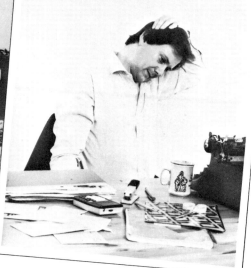

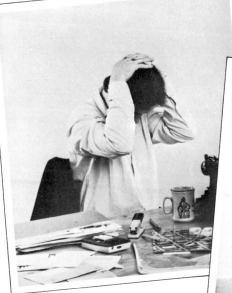

2 RIGHT **Breathe in. As you breathe out, drop your head to the left and place your left arm across your head. Keep your chin in and let your jaw hang open. Hold until you feel a gentle stretch. Breathe in and lift the head. Repeat on the right side.**

Strengthening Exercises

Your aerobic exercise is all-important in improving the efficiency of your heart and lungs, which is the key to physical fitness. The exercises that follow are designed to complement that improvement by building up muscle strength and increasing fitness overall. Like aerobic exercise, they are equally as suitable for women as for men – and they won't produce bulging muscles but an improved body shape, without flab or paunches.

By combining the home exercises with an aerobic exercise, the level of fitness can be increased. They should be done twice a week, on days that you are not doing your aerobic exercise, although if you also play squash or another sport once a week, you may prefer to consider that as a substitute. The exercises are again graded into beginners, intermediate and advanced levels, and for those who are already quite fit and wish to train more seriously, there are additional exercises using weights.

The strengthening exercises done on their own after you have finished the 12-week course will help to maintain fitness, and they make a good starting point from which to repeat the programme in the future.

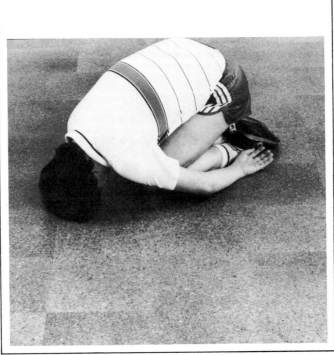

The rest position, curled in a ball, to follow the series of exercises.
"Neil had no trouble with this one." – *Catherine*

The first run. What have I got myself into? I don't really want to step outside into the cold air. I'd much rather stay in bed and listen to the radio, have a hot bath and get to work in my usual unrushed way. Why, oh why, did I agree to all this effort? I feel enormous resentment as I pull on my new tracksuit and new, hugely expensive shoes, which I am told are an essential.

The front door slams behind me

It might as well be the gates of Pentonville or Sing Sing. I feel like a condemned man. The whole idea is stupid – I feel stupid, I probably look stupid. I walk out of sight of the house and self-consciously break into a trot. I head for the local recreation ground, which is not very big and is grassed. Already my breathing is laboured and I spew condensed breath into the dank March air. The only visible sign of life is a mangy dog which gives me a pitying glance as I run by. I look at my watch and am astonished to see that only four minutes have passed since I left the house – it feels like 40.

I complete one circuit of the park and begin another

My legs are like stone weights and it takes considerable effort to pick them up out of the lush grass. The park, I now notice, is built on a severe slope. I decide to get the circuit over as quickly as possible and attack the pace – with the result that my lungs burn and my heart races. I head out of the park and make for the house but, remembering earlier advice not to strain, slow down into a walk. I reach home and the coughing starts – an explosion of bile and phlegm. Only the hot bath is consolation.

The second run

This is as unpleasant an experience as the first run, but I accept that I must persevere and do my best to stick to my plan: to run on Mondays, Wednesdays and Fridays – with the prospect of absolutely no exercise on the week-ends. On Tuesdays and Thursdays I intend either to play squash or do exercises at home.

My first running effort, pathetic as it was, has given me guidelines to follow. I managed then to be on the go for eight minutes – which I am told is hardly aerobic. It may not be aerobic but it is quite enough for me at the moment. My lungs and heart are unused to such enforced labour; any more of it and I would be in definite pain.

So again I run for eight minutes and again I end up coughing. I am told that this is because I am running too fast. I must try to slow down on the next outing.

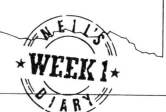

The third run

It is a foul day, rain and wind, yet I am still out here pounding and panting. For the first time I feel a hint of satisfaction coming over me – I have at least had the discipline to get out of bed. Admittedly, I had a good bribe: hot tea and a hotter bath will be waiting when I return in 8 to 10 minutes.

Lungs, heart, legs and various unknown organs make their objections felt as they are once again diverted from their usual early morning routine of civilised sloth. Here I am in the park in the name of greater fitness and rectitude, and the bile is rising, leaving a nasty metallic taste in the mouth. I regret that wine of yesterday evening; I am sure that it is impeding my progress. This time when I reach home, I don't cough. I must be doing something right.

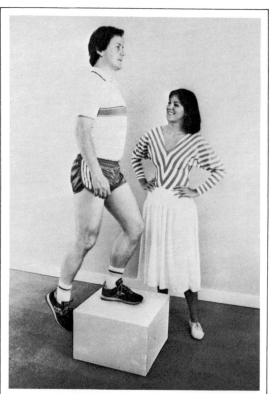

Strengthening Exercises – Beginners

If you are very unfit, progress through the 10 exercises here and on pages 50-54 at your own pace. Once you have become fitter, start building up the number of times you can do all the exercises against the clock. To determine how many repetitions of each exercise that you should do, count the number of times that you can do each exercise over a period of 60 seconds, working as fast as possible. Rest after each exercise.

To work against the clock, the complete circuit of exercises should be done in quick succession, repeating each exercise the number of times that you were able to do it in one minute. Rest after doing this, then do the complete circuit again but at half the number of repetitions. The aim is to see how many times you are able to do the complete circuit in this way within a period of 10 minutes. Once you are fitter, you can increase the time period up to 20 minutes.

1 LEFT *Step-ups:* **Use a solid box or bench and step up on to it with the right leg, straightening the knee as you bring the left leg up beside it. Step down with the right leg and then the left. Repeat, leading with the left leg. To be done in a continuous rhythm.**

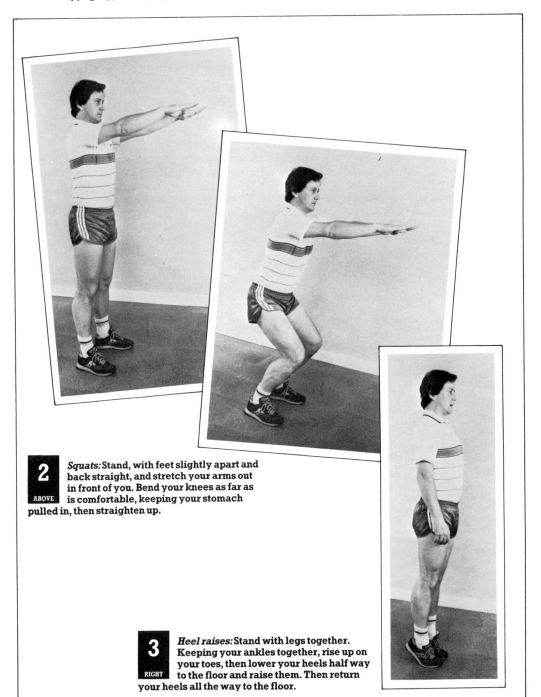

2 **ABOVE** *Squats:* Stand, with feet slightly apart and back straight, and stretch your arms out in front of you. Bend your knees as far as is comfortable, keeping your stomach pulled in, then straighten up.

3 **RIGHT** *Heel raises:* Stand with legs together. Keeping your ankles together, rise up on your toes, then lower your heels half way to the floor and raise them. Then return your heels all the way to the floor.

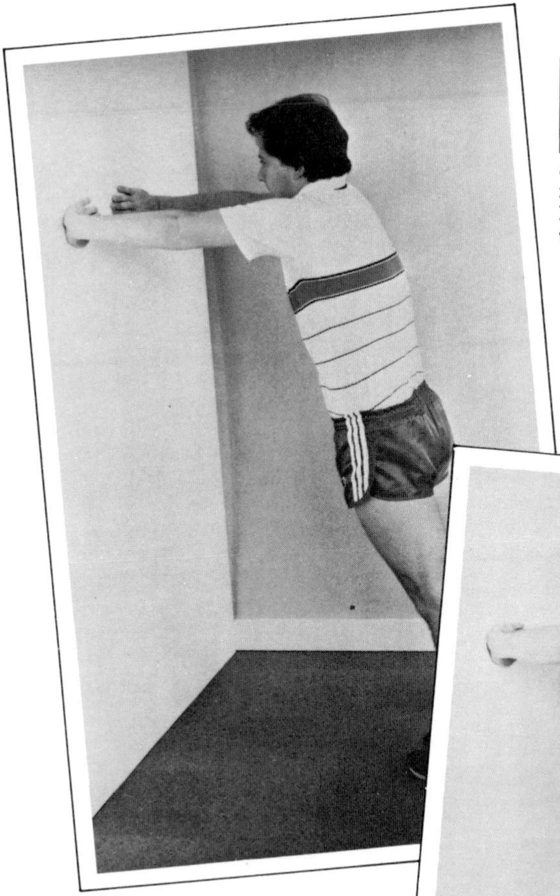

4

LEFT & BELOW

Press offs: Lean hands against a wall, fingers pointing towards each other, with your body slanting forwards in a straight line and arms at full stretch. Bend your arms, moving your body forwards in a straight line, and push off strongly, straightening the arms.

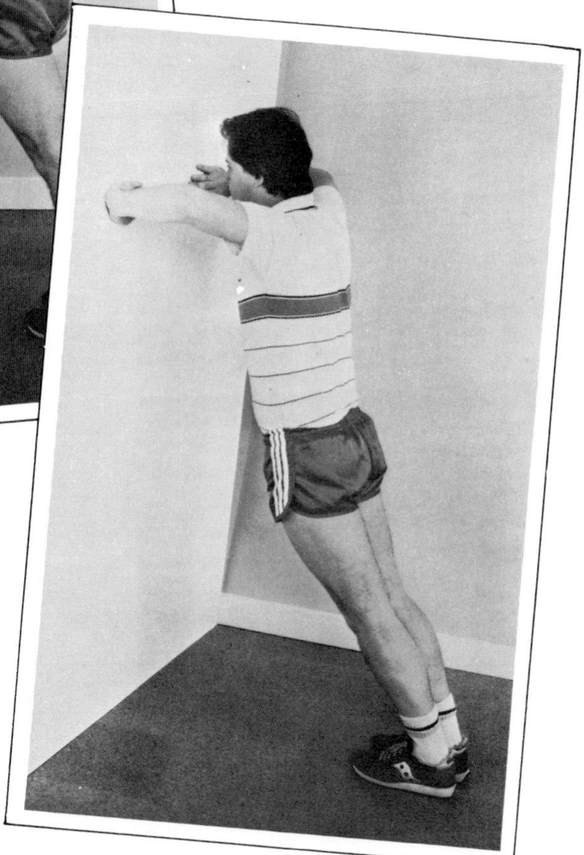

NEIL'S WEEK 2 DIARY

Three circuits of the little park completed and I am no closer to enjoying the experience. My mangy friend is back and looks astonished to see me again. Feelings of self-consciousness now have all but gone. It was like that when I had to wear short trousers at school – everyone else did, so the shame was somehow reduced. But there are no other joggers in the park. I must think about changing location: this place is boring, uneven and, I now realise, saps the energy because the grass is wet and long.

A companion for me

My good friend Sophie hears on the grapevine that I am to be seen running around the parish in a tracksuit. *"Would I like to join her for a jog?"* Indicating that, for scientific reasons, my outings must be gentle, I accept. She is fitter than I am and has more stamina. She is married to an extremely sporting man who does not allow a day to pass without dragging her on to the squash or tennis court or insisting on a quick five-mile run.

This is the first time that I have been joined on a run by a fellow human being. It makes a lot of difference. Although I have so far only managed to run for 10 minutes without a break, I now somehow manage about 18 minutes jogging around the streets of Notting Hill. I resolve to find company on my runs again.

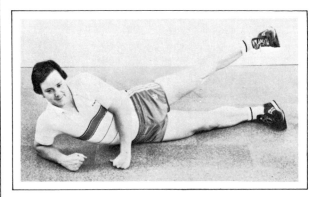

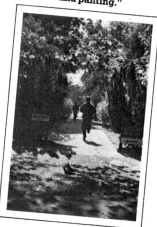

"Still out here pounding and panting."

5 **ABOVE** *Leg lifts:* Lie on your side resting on your elbow, knees facing straight forward. Lift your top leg, holding your stomach in, and lower leg half way down, then lift and lower all the way. Repeat with the other leg.

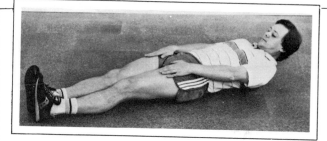

6
LEFT
Sit ups: Lie on your back, hands resting on thighs. Lift head and shoulders just enough to look at your toes, keeping legs straight and sliding hands down towards your knees. (Do not sit right up.) Keep stomach held in and push small of back into the floor as you lift up. Lower.

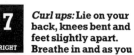

7
RIGHT
Curl ups: Lie on your back, knees bent and feet slightly apart. Breathe in and as you breathe out reach forwards for your knees, pushing lower back into the floor and sucking stomach muscles in. Lower.

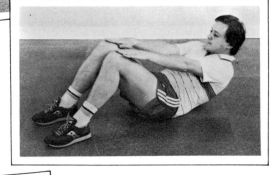

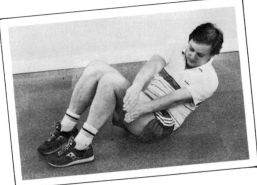

8
LEFT
Diagonal curl ups: Lie on your back, feet slightly apart and knees bent. Breathe in and as you breathe out, reach to the outside of your right knee, keeping your stomach held in. Lower, and repeat to the left.

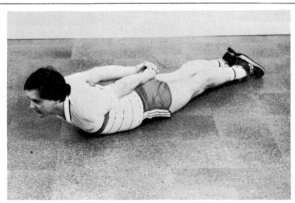

 9
LEFT
Back lifts: Lie on your front and clasp your hands above your bottom, keeping your elbows straight. Lift your head and shoulders. Hold, and lower.

10
BELOW
Diagonal back lifts: Lie on your front and stretch your arms above your head. Breathe in and as you breathe out, lift your right arm and left leg, keeping stomach held in. Lower and repeat with left arm and right leg.

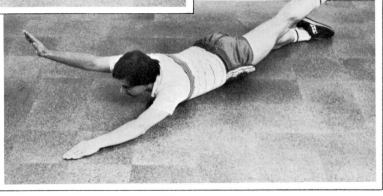

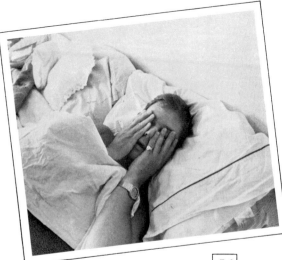

"It takes a firm will to get out on the streets . . . Bed is never more comfortable and the prospect of a run never more unattractive."

INTERMEDIATE

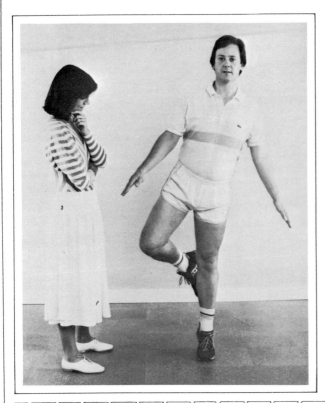

Strengthening Exercises – Intermediate

The 10 exercises here and on pages 56-60 should be done against the clock for a period of 10 minutes or up to 20 minutes. To determine the number of repetitions of each exercise that you should do when working against the clock, first do each exercise as fast as possible for one minute, resting after each.

To work against the clock, the complete circuit of exercises should be done in quick succession, repeating each exercise the number of times that you were able to do it in one minute. Rest after doing this, then start the complete circuit again but doing half the number of repetitions of each exercise. The aim is to see how many times that you can do the complete circuit in this way within your specified time limit.

1 *Heel raises:* Stand on one leg and bend the other leg up behind you, using your arms to balance yourself. Go up on to the ball of your foot, lower the heel towards the floor and push up. Repeat on the other leg.

I have serious doubts that I will be able to sustain the course to the end. I cheer myself with the realisation that at the end of this, my third week, I will have completed a quarter of the programme.

It takes a firm will to get out on the streets when you wake to hear the rain beating on the window. Bed is never more comfortable and the prospect of a run never more unattractive. But, although I have not admitted this to Catherine, I am beginning to share the joggers' feelings of self-satisfaction. You can consider all the good that you are doing yourself while the rest of the population is slowly killing itself over its breakfasts of fatty bacon and eggs. Maybe I am not yet a convert but I no longer think of joggers as self-righteous hypochondriacs with nothing better to do than frighten old ladies in the park as they pound down the paths in absurd clothing.

NEIL'S WEEK 3 DIARY

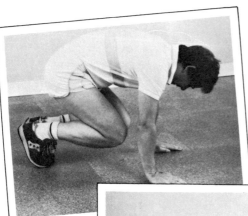

2

LEFT & BELOW

Alternate leg thrusts: Crouch on all fours, taking your weight on your hands. Kick each leg out behind you alternately.

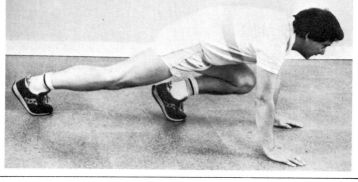

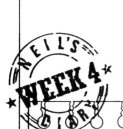

I join forces with Hetty, who wears a T-shirt that shamelessly advertises her book *Dieting Makes You Fat*. Hetty is not fat and she is a professional jogger so she is useful to someone like me who knows nothing about the technique of running. It appears that I do not have an economical style so I exhaust myself more quickly than I otherwise would. I also must learn to pace myself: I am too quick out of the blocks, which leaves me struggling at the end of a run.

Astonishing progress
I go out again with Hetty, who shows me a course of nearly three miles in Hyde Park. We run from Bayswater to Kensington Gore, around Kensington House, along to the Albert Memorial, turn left at the Serpentine and back along the fourth side of the "square" to our start. It takes us 21 minutes – a speed of about 7mph. To think that less than a month ago I could only manage a run of eight minutes is astonishing to me.

INTERMEDIATE

3
BELOW & RIGHT
Squat jumps: Squat, touching the floor with your finger tips. Spring upwards as high as you can, and touch the floor again with your hands when you come down. To be done in a continuous movement.

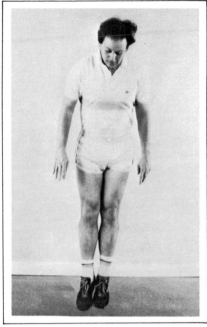

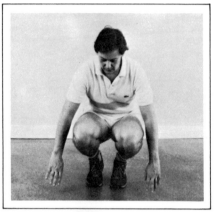

4
BELOW
Leg thrusts: Crouch on all fours, taking your weight on your hands, and kick both legs together straight out behind you. Keep bending and straightening in a continuous movement.

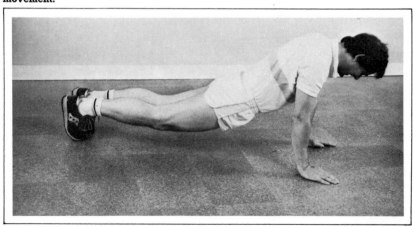

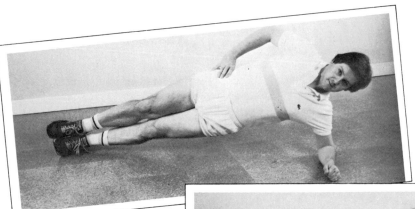

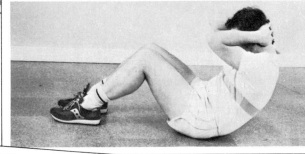

5 **ABOVE** *Side lifts:* Lie on your side, body in a straight line and resting on your elbow. Lift up the whole of your trunk by pushing down on your elbow and lower arm. Lower and repeat.

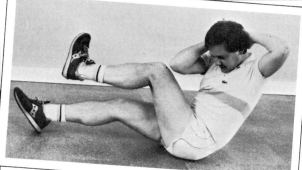

6 **ABOVE** *Curl ups:* Lie on your back with knees bent, feet flat on the floor. Clasp your hands behind your head and lift your head and shoulders to try to touch your knees with your elbows. Lower back slowly, keeping stomach held in throughout.

7 **ABOVE** *Diagonal curl ups:* Lie flat on your back with your hands clasped behind your head. Lift your left knee towards your chest, bringing your head and shoulders forwards to touch the left knee with your right elbow. Lower back slowly, keeping stomach held in throughout. Repeat, touching your right knee with your left elbow.

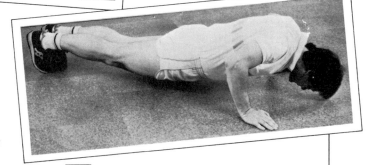

NEIL'S WEEK 5 DIARY

The change of scene has made a major difference to my mental attitude. The little park was uninteresting, and all I had for company was a scruffy old dog. Here in Hyde Park I have many things to keep my mind occupied. Spring is around the corner. The bulbs are forcing themselves out of the ground, the crocuses are already in bloom. I am beginning to feel a camaraderie with my fellow joggers. All is wonderful.

I join Hetty again, who suggests a slightly longer run. I agree. For the first time I feel that I am able to run faster than her but because we are doing a longer circuit, I restrict myself. This might be a good sign – could it mean that I am beginning to find the runs enjoyable? Surely not! Other joggers provide diversion. I imagine that one very old man is doing his best to keep fit for a young lover. The effort leaves him without the energy to make the customary greeting to other early morning runners.

Setting some kind of record

I tackle the circuit with determination and, despite my earlier intentions, make a sprint for home – just to see if I can do it. I can, but I am so exhausted at the end that I collapse panting on a fence. The sweat pours off me, and my pulse is exploding. But the feeling is rather nice – is this the joggers' addiction that I've heard about?

I return home to tell proudly of my achievement: I completed the course in my fastest time ever – 18 minutes. Our adviser Vivian Grisogono telephones and is far from congratulatory. Was I being stupidly competitive? Was I still enjoying the trees, the daffodils? I admit that I was obsessed with bettering my time. I am duly admonished.

8 LEFT

Press ups: Lie on your stomach, with hands underneath your shoulders and fingers facing forwards, feet slightly apart. Press up on your hands, breathing in, and lower as you breathe out.

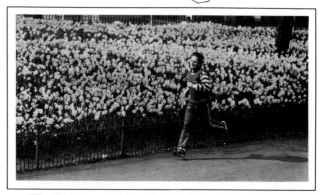

"The flowers are in bloom in Hyde Park. All is wonderful."

9

BELOW

Back lifts: Lie on your stomach with arms outstretched at shoulder level. Lift your arms, shoulders and head plus your legs off the floor, and hold. Lower. Clench your bottom as you lift up.

10

BOTTOM

Leg lifts: Lie on your stomach, resting your forehead on your hands, placed on top of each other. Breathe in and as you breathe out, clench your bottom and lift your legs off the floor. Separate and bring together your legs in the air, in a scissor movement.

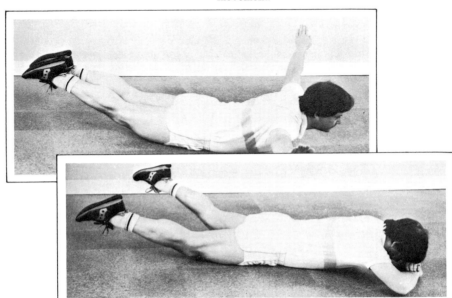

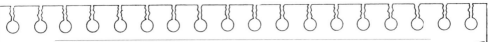

It's now nearly the half-way mark in the programme and, just as I'm feeling so much fitter, I find myself with a problem. On my 20-minute runs this week, I found it hard to get around the course. I began to hate the slightly uphill final straight, which appeared to have no end. It is long and the trees alongside the path are planted in regimented lines that seem designed to produce weariness. I tried counting the trees but I gave up after the fifteenth.

Although, as I am constantly reminded, the pleasure principle is the philosophy of the programme, there are times when a run is not pleasurable. Everyone has off days when for some reason the body does not respond to the demands placed upon it. These set-backs are, I am told, to be expected. They are there to be overcome.

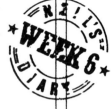

ADVANCED

Strengthening Exercises – Advanced

The 10 exercises following should be done against the clock for 10 minutes or up to 20 minutes. See page 55 for working out the number of repetitions of each exercise that you should aim for.

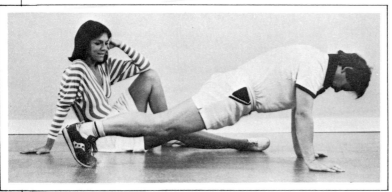

1 LEFT *Squat thrusts:* Crouch on all fours, taking your weight on your hands. Kick both legs straight out behind you and keep bending and straightening them in a continuous movement.

NEIL'S WEEK 7 DIARY

On the advice of Hetty, I break my no exercise on weekends rule and join up with a rather serious looking group of runners who meet on Saturdays at the Serpentine. What is in store is my longest and hardest run of the training programme but I am initially fooled by one of the runners who says that I will find the run a doddle. After preliminary stretch exercises demonstrated by a rubber-bodied teacher (I can get nowhere near an imitation), we all set off around the Serpentine. I have done this two- to three-mile run before and it is true that it is a doddle. However, I learn during it that this is just the "family run" when everyone potters around making polite conversation. The main run comes later – round the perimeter of Hyde Park, a distance of about seven miles. That will make a total of nearly ten.

Triumph of the will

I feel that it is time to go home after the first run but I am made to feel ashamed at giving up now: the next run should be within my capability. I agree to try, and hope that I will not conk out outside the Albert Hall. I manage the first quarter of the course and, rather to my surprise, feel able to continue. Past half-way I feel proud enough to call it a day, but my strong companion asks whether I would not feel a greater sense of satisfaction if I went just a little bit further.

I completed the course – and the sense of satisfaction was very gratifying. I had run further than ever before and I did not collapse in a heap at the end. It proved that I could tackle longer distances if the spirit was willing. I had run 10 miles, whereas a month and a half ago I had been unable to do much more than a mile. Improvement was taking place.

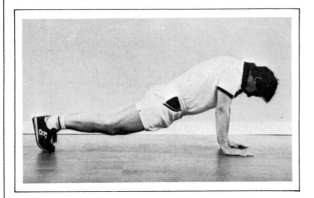

3
RIGHT
Bench jumps: Stand with your legs on either side of a box, bench or other object about 18 inches high. With arms outstretched, jump up, kicking your heels together in the air, and land in the starting position. (Use a cardboard rather than wooden box if you're concerned about where you might land!)

2
THIS PAGE
Burpees: This is similar to a squat thrust but with an intervening jump. Begin, as before, in the crouch position, taking your weight on your hands and kick both legs straight out behind you (above). When you return to the squat position (below), jump straight up as far as you can (right). Return to the squat position and repeat the whole movement.

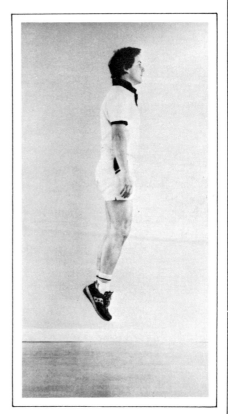

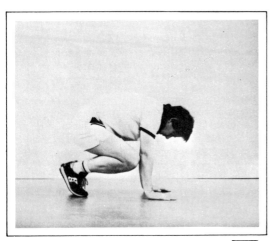

ADVANCED

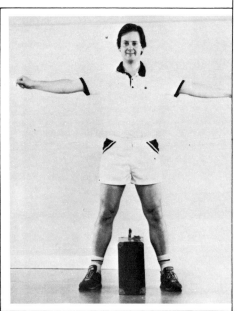

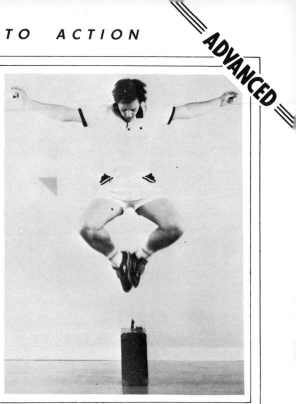

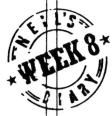

I consolidate the great effort of Saturday with two 20-minute runs and face my fear of the long uphill finishing stretch. I find the problem can be overcome simply by steadier pacing and not being as competitive with myself. At the end of the run I feel satisfied that I have completed the three miles in the allotted time and I am not cross that I have not broken my earlier record. This, then, is the pleasure principle at work.

I come across an apposite quotation from Roger Bannister: *"Running has given me a glimpse of the greatest freedom that a man can ever know, because it results in the simultaneous liberation of both body and mind."* It is true, although I would never have thought it several weeks ago.

Equanimity
Running is different, I am beginning to discover, from my favourite indoor game, squash. After a good run, the whole body pulses gently and literally glows with health. (Friends are telling me that my cheeks have lost that night-club pallor.) A game of squash can have the same effect but because it is so intensely competitive (every point must be fought if ultimate victory is desired), losing can leave one feeling cheated or downright annoyed. This, says my exercise guru, is negative and stressful. I am not sure about that but I have tried to run for fun and not get into any races with fitter friends.

NEIL'S WEEK 9 DIARY

Running this week is a joy. The flowers are in bloom and I marvel at the trees, which are loaded down with blossom. The only hazards on the paths are randy ducks oblivious of flying feet.

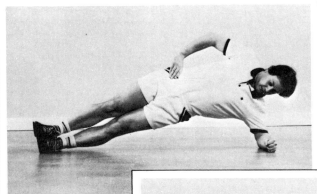

4 LEFT

Side lifts: **Lie on your side, body in a straight line and resting on your elbow. Lift up the whole of your trunk by pushing down on your elbow and lower arm. Lower.**

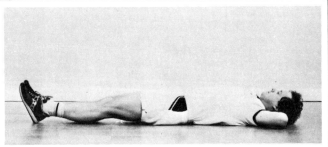

5 ABOVE & RIGHT

Curl ups: **Lie on your back, with hands clasped behind your head. Bend your knees and lift both legs, bringing your head and shoulders forwards to touch your knees with your elbows. Breathe in as you lie flat and out as you lift up. Lower yourself down slowly.**

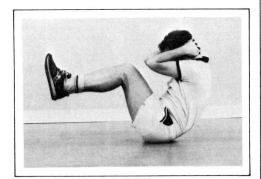

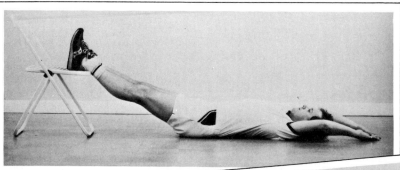

6 ABOVE & RIGHT *Chair curl ups:* Lie on your back, resting your feet and ankles on a chair seat and stretching your arms above your head. Breathe in. As you breathe out, lift your upper body, keeping your legs straight and stomach held in, and reach forwards to touch your ankles with your fingers.

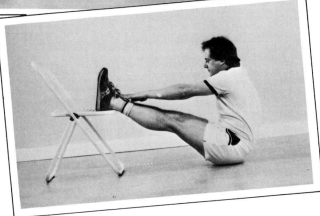

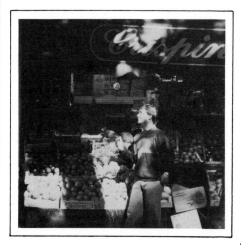

"Running this week is a joy. Fruit can fly as well as my feet."

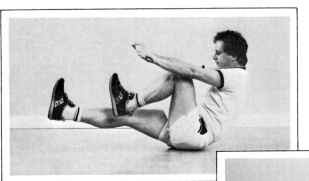

7

LEFT & BELOW

Curl ups with belt: Holding a belt taut between your hands, lie on your back with your arms straight out behind your head. Lift your arms, head and shoulders, and bend your left knee, sliding the belt under it and then straightening the leg. Reverse the movement. Repeat, sliding the belt under your right knee.

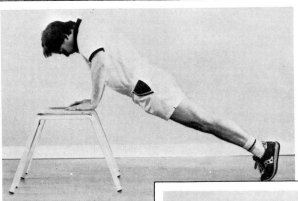

8

LEFT & BELOW

Press ups between chairs: Place two chairs or stools about a shoulder's width apart. Lean a hand on each chair and stretch body out in a straight line behind, toes on floor. Start with the arms straight, then bend them and lower chest to seat level; straighten arms, bend them and lower chest to below seat.

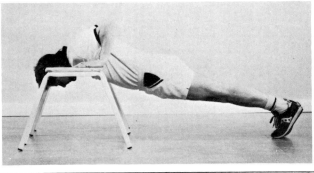

ADVANCED

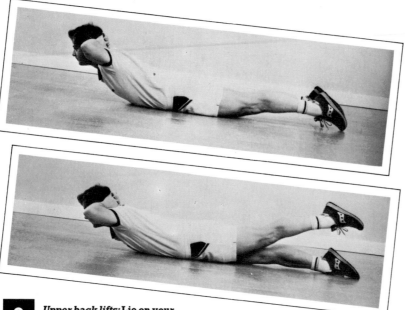

9

TOP

Upper back lifts: Lie on your stomach, hands clasped behind your head. Lift your head, shoulders and back, keeping feet on floor, and hold for a count of three. Lower gently.

10

ABOVE

Back and leg lifts: Lie on your stomach, hands clasped behind your head. Lift your head and shoulders together with your right leg. Lower and lift again with your left leg. Repeat in quick succession.

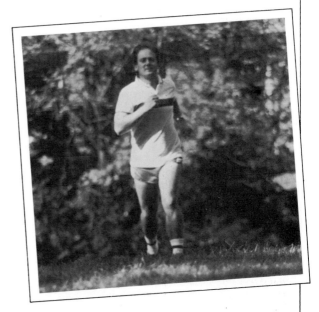

"The long uphill stretch . . . and I am now enjoying running. What an admission!"

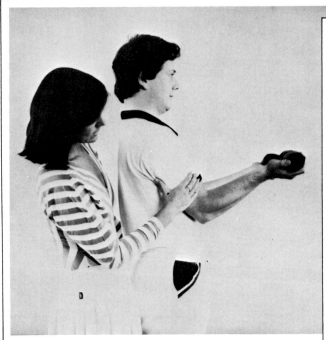

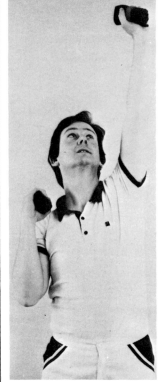

1 ABOVE *Arms:* Stand (or sit) holding a weight in each hand, arms by your sides. Bring your arms up, drawing the weights into your chest, and lower in one continuous movement.

2 RIGHT *Upper back and arms:* Stand (or sit) holding a weight in each hand at shoulder level. Push one arm straight up above your head and as you lower it, push up the other arm.

Working with Weights

Weight training improves muscle strength and can be used to work on particular muscle groups. Weights should not be used by a beginner, nor by people with high blood pressure unless they are professionally monitored.

The weight exercises here are simple and use light, 2lb, weights. You can buy these weights at sports shops or alternatively you can use 2lb bags of sugar or beans (enclosed in a stronger bag).

The eight exercises can be added to the intermediate or advanced programme to further increase strength, or one or more of them used to build up a specific area, such as the arms if they are weak. Start off by doing 10 repetitions of each exercise and build up slowly to do three sets of 10. *Stop the exercise if you begin to feel any pain.*

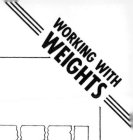

NEIL'S ★ WEEK 10 ★ DIARY

The end of the plan is in sight and I am now enjoying running. What an admission. I ring up my super-fit friend, the one who jogs in downtown Baghdad, and suggest a gentle run along the canal bank. He accepts and we go off on a run that turns into a mini-marathon. Half an hour stretches to an hour and we complete seven miles with little bursts of sprint thrown in. It does not bother me that I am out-sprinted. It shows that there is capacity for me to get even fitter, but I do not wish to over-achieve. For the first time since school I believe that I am properly fit, and I have little desire to train to exacting competition standard. This is recreation.

3
BOTTOM & BELOW

Arms and shoulders: Stand (or sit) and stretch out your arms at shoulder level. Squeeze your shoulder blades together, then raise your arms and lower them to shoulder height.

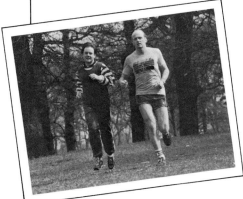

"My super-fit friend, the Baghdad jogger."

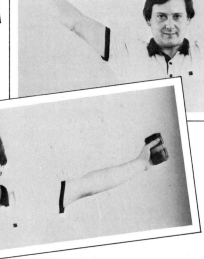

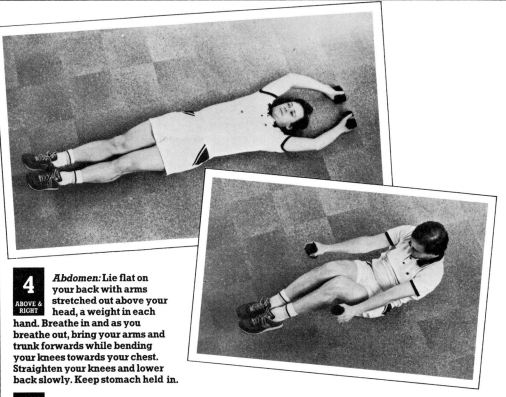

4

ABOVE & RIGHT

Abdomen: Lie flat on your back with arms stretched out above your head, a weight in each hand. Breathe in and as you breathe out, bring your arms and trunk forwards while bending your knees towards your chest. Straighten your knees and lower back slowly. Keep stomach held in.

5

BELOW

Side of legs: Place a weight around your right ankle and lie on your left side. Lift up your right leg, keeping your knee facing straight forwards. Lower the leg half way towards the floor, raise it and then lower all the way. Repeat with other leg.

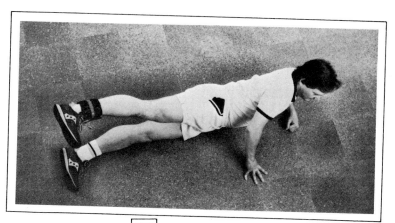

WORKING WITH WEIGHTS

I feel ready to submit myself to the critical gaze of our professional sports adviser, Tony, who suggests a run around Hyde Park. While I feel able to run this distance, I have my doubts about being assessed by the knowing Tony. Off we set, at a pace a little faster than I would choose. All is well at first but suddenly I feel the strain. Tony is happily chatting. I concentrate on the pace and the style of running – letting the hands drop to the side helps. I remember one of Hetty's running tips and startle Tony with a shouted exhalation of air – a trick to keep one's energy up. Now the pace seems a little more civilised but I look forward to the end of the circuit. As if to indicate that I am not in a race, I drop the pace within sight of the finishing line and walk the final 100 yards.

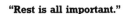

It seems that I pass the test

Some months later I learned that Tony had been playing with me like a fish on a line. He had been picking up and dropping the pace to test my ability to respond. Not knowing what he was up to, I simply kept his right shoulder in sight.

NEIL'S WEEK 11 DIARY

"Rest is all important."

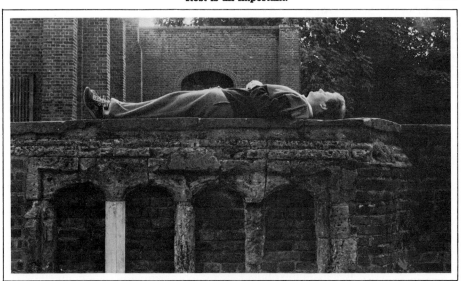

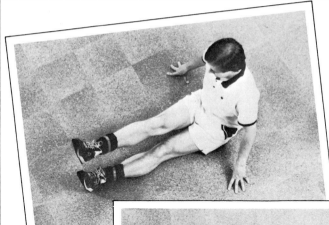

6 **LEFT** *Front of legs:* Place a weight around each ankle and sit with legs stretched out straight and back upright. Keeping your knees straight, lift up one leg and lower it slowly. Repeat with other leg.

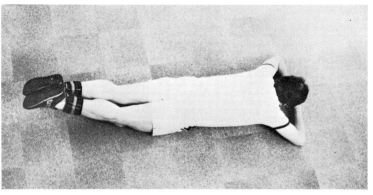

7 **ABOVE** *Legs and buttocks:* Place a weight around each ankle and lie on your stomach, resting your head on your hands. Clench your buttocks and lift both legs off the floor. Hold for a count of three, and lower.

8 **BELOW** *Upper back and arms:* Lie on your stomach, arms stretched out above your head and with a weight in each hand. Lift arms, shoulders and back from the floor and hold for a count of three. Lower slowly.

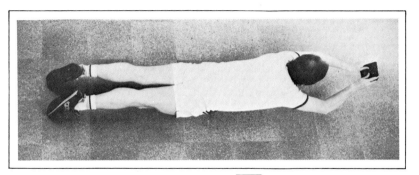

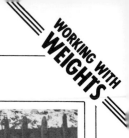

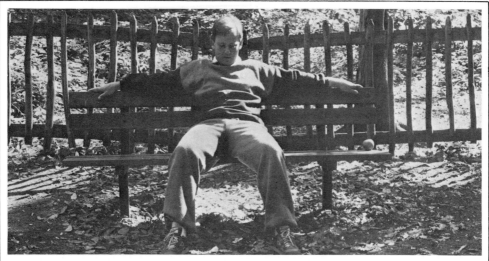

**"The end of a good run . . .
and the whole body pulses gently."**

I may be no long-distance runner – Tony had referred to my sprinter's legs once or twice as we circuited Hyde Park – but now at the end of the three months I think that I have achieved my desired target. My stomach has vanished. I am back to a size 32-inch waist. My complexion has improved. I no longer wake up every morning feeling awful. I feel free of the petty anxieties of daily living.

At the start of this plan I chuckled at the words of Noel Coward who said: *"Exercise is the most awful illusion. The secret is a lot of aspirins and marrons glacés."* But he was wrong. Running has made a difference – an enormous difference according to friends, who have commented on the change in my appearance. I have a new sense of well-being.

I sound like a convert

All the same, I can only point out the benefits. The early stages were harder than I thought they would be and I was in danger at any moment of giving up the whole idea. If I had, I would never have known what I stood to gain.

Next week I journey to the sports laboratory at Birmingham University to let the machines decide scientifically if I have made the progress that I think that I have. It will be a day of judgement and, despite all the work, I am nervous at the prospect of being trussed-up on their unforgiving treadmill.

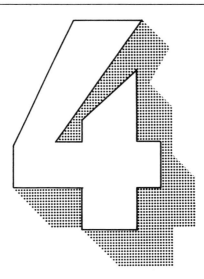

Eating and Drinking into Shape

THERE'S A GOOD CHANCE that the reason your man – or you – decided to get into shape was, simply, fat – he looked, and was, overweight. There's an even higher chance that, overweight or not, his eating and drinking habits were a major source of concern. The point of our 12-week programme is to establish a healthier life-style as pleasurably as possible, and the answer to that is not to go on a stringent diet or to stop eating what you enjoy and to cut out the booze altogether. What is needed is a change of emphasis in eating and drinking habits, to go along with the exercise course and not ruin all the good work being done there.

Remember that if being overweight is the problem, regular vigorous exercise, not calorie-counting, is the most effective way to take off fat and keep it off. According to recent research, exercise boosts the body's metabolic rate to the extent that you can even eat more, rather than less, and still lose weight. A crash diet, on the other hand, is not only no pleasure but rarely succeeds. Eighty per cent of people who go on a diet put back on within a year the weight that

they have lost. All that they have done is impose on themselves an unnecessarily strict regime which probably deprived the body of adequate nourishment while it lasted.

It is time to stop stringent diets and become fitter without neurotic recourse to bathroom scales at every turn. Weigh yourself at the beginning of the 12-week programme, then once a month thereafter. Do not judge your fitness by the scales. If you began the course overweight, you will certainly see a difference but muscles weigh more as they are developed and some people may not show as much weight loss as they expected. The new, trim shape, though, will be obvious; the tape-measure can prove it.

For our shape-up plan, there are no rules about what you should eat and drink. It is recognised that people will find themselves in pubs, restaurants and parties during the 12 weeks, and tips are given to help you get through these difficult pastures. It is not suggested that you starve yourself or become a vegetarian, vegan or vitamin fanatic. Nor is it suggested that you wave the flag for the temperance movement for three months; the flesh being weak, that would probably result only in broken promises and a hangover. What we do suggest is that you aim to eat foods that are energy-giving, not particularly rich in calories, and a delight to eat; and that you cut down your alcohol intake. This might mean giving up chips, sugar and beer, sticking to low-calorie soft drinks and eating in a more responsible way – not drowning your strawberries in clotted cream or having buttered crumpets for tea every weekend.

In the following pages, the qualities of various foods and the medical opinions about diet are outlined, to give you a general idea of what to eat – and what to avoid – to benefit your health. It is up to you whether you follow the latest medical opinion, which incidentally is always on the move, or reject it out of hand and continue to fry eggs in lard for breakfast and over-salt everything on your plate.

The food debate

There has recently been a spate of publications about diet and health that have dramatically changed the way that we look at food. In the old days the inch war was what mattered. Now, it is evidently all right again to eat but *what* we are eating may be killing us. It is no longer the size of our hips that is of overriding interest but the shape of our hearts and bowels and lungs. Have we lost one obsession only to gain another? The 1980s could be witnessing a new neurosis called the "public fear of food". It was enough that eating used to make you fat; now we are having to face that it kills.

Margaret Flynn, Professor of Family and Community Medicine at the University of Missouri-Columbia, has recognised the new fear and points out that for every argument that a food is seriously detrimental to our health, there is a counter-argument. "Some believe it will be a long time before we have iron-clad evidence for a connection between diet, heart disease and cancer, so we cannot sit back and wait; we must recommend dietary changes to lessen risk. Other researchers look at the same basic scientific data and are emphatic that the information is inadequate for recommendations to drastically change what people choose to eat."

The Health Education Council reports that heart disease is the biggest single killer in Britain today and it estimates that four out of every ten men will suffer from some form of heart disease by the time that they are 65 years old. A major contributor to heart disease, we are told, is a high level of cholesterol in the blood, which is linked with a high consumption of saturated fats.

In their 1984 report on diet and cardiovascular disease, the Committee on Medical Aspects of Food Policy (COMA) maintains that if you eat less fat and do not increase your sugar and salt consumption, you will "probably" reduce the risk of heart disease. It concludes that "the prevention of cardiovascular disease by dietary and other means is a sufficiently important subject to merit on-going review".

One recommendation for avoiding early death from heart disease is to eat more fish and less red meat, something that the American Heart Association has long advocated. A recent survey

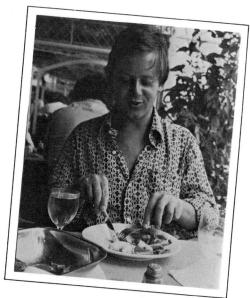

"I tested my will power against the skill of the chef. Sometimes I didn't win."

in Holland of 852 middle-aged Dutchmen found that the incidence of fatal heart disease was more than 50 per cent lower among men who regularly ate fish than among those who ate no fish at all. This was despite the fact that the fish-eaters consumed more meat than the non-fish-eaters and had a higher proportion of cholesterol intake in their diet. The Dutch study concluded that modest amounts of seafood – one or two fish dishes a week – "may be of value in the prevention of coronary heart disease". Some scientists say that it is too early to say whether the theories about fish are valid; they could be the beginning of a break-through or another fashionable dead-end.

Alarmingly, epidemiologists tell us that 30 to 60 per cent of cancers have dietary factors as a contributory cause. Eating habits in general have come under scrutiny and Western man's diet found to be unbalanced and potentially harmful. Not only do we eat too much fat and meat (the two often go together) but too much sugar, which has no nutritional value, and too much salt. Cancer of the colon has been linked with lack of fibre in our diet, and hypertension – high blood pressure – with excessive salt intake. The latter theory has been around since the beginning of the twentieth century and is now widely accepted, though the mechanism whereby salt could lead to the development of hypertension has not yet been established.

Taking a balanced view

New, worrying theories about diet are reaching us all the time and the only sensible course of action is to take note of them but not become neurotic about it. If your hostess cooks with cream all the way through a meal, don't start imagining that you are going to have a heart seizure. Our health is the sum total of what we eat, think and do, our genetic inheritance and the foundations laid in childhood. It can take as long as 30 years to see the detrimental effects of, say, too much consumption of sugar. What we can try to do now is reset the balance to keep the risk factors down. Remember that if you worry unduly about your health, you are increasing stress – a contributing factor, some say a major

one, to ill health. The health of your mind and emotions is of equal importance to that of your digestive system and arteries.

Choose the middle way: learn a bit more about nutrition and aim to reduce fat, sugar and salt intake, which are the three aspects of diet that the health experts broadly agree on. The fact that the body needs a food intake of 70 to 80 per cent carbohydrate, 20 to 30 per cent fat and 8 to 10 per cent protein is of academic interest. If you follow the general guidelines here about eating and drinking, your body will be getting all that it needs to maintain a healthy system.

Guidelines for a balanced diet

- Try not to eat meat more than once a day and keep the portion to about 4 oz.

- Cut down fat consumption; switch to low-fat dairy products, take small helpings of foods containing cream and butter.

- Avoid cakes, sweets, biscuits and all foods high in sugar; use artificial sweeteners in drinks.

- Eat more vegetables, raw foods, salads and fruits.

- Eat wholemeal bread.

- Forego the bowls of salted nuts and crisps, and watch your action with the salt cellar.

- Restrict the amount of coffee you drink.

- Cut down on alcohol.

- Eat a sensible breakfast.

- Don't have snacks between meals.

- Regulate your meals during the day so that if you have a heavy lunch, eat a light dinner and if lunch was a snack, eat dinner early.

Meat and protein

Even those who know little about nutrition are aware that man must get his protein. It is vital for body maintenance, i.e. tissue building and repair. In the West, we tend to get our protein through animal products rather than vegetables and grains. Animal proteins – from meat, eggs and dairy products – are known as complete proteins because they provide a balance of essential amino acids – the bricks from which proteins are made. (Of the 22 amino acids needed by the body, eight cannot be made in the body but must be obtained from protein foods.) Vegetable proteins are known as incomplete proteins because they do not provide the full balance of amino acids, although by mixing the diet with other protein sources, such as nuts and soya, a vegetarian can ensure a full balance without recourse to meat and animal products.

Many people would consider that they had not eaten a good dinner without having meat but to judge by the amount of meat consumed in an average Westerner's diet, one would think we were trying to make up for structural damage to our bodies. There is nothing wrong with meat and a lot right with it, not least its taste, but we tend to eat too much of it. Meat contains fat and, in the forms that we frequently eat meat, it contains a high proportion of fat. Sausages, for example, are as much as 72 per cent fat. Much better is to increase our intake of vegetable proteins.

It is not suggested that you cut meat out of your diet. As Tom Stobart, author of *The Cook's Encyclopedia*, says: "Surely one of the most depressing statements ever made is that the world could support a population of 16,000 million people if everyone ate soya beans instead of meat. An acre of these beans can keep a moderately active man alive (but not necessarily contented) for 2200 days, while the same acre would keep him for only 75 days if he lived on beef."

The advice is to switch the balance of the meal away from meat to fish, vegetables, rice and grains, pasta and salads, and to reduce similarly the amount of dairy products you eat. Try to restrict yourself to three eggs a week, for example. The days of the half-pound steak are over, for financial as well as health reasons. In Tom Stobart's words, "The daily requirement of protein for an adult would be satisfied by about half a pound of meat or chicken per day, with no protein coming from any other source, but most people in Europe and America get their requirement from a mixed diet and 4 to 5 ounces of meat per day is enough."

Fats

Fats, like disasters, come in threes: polyunsaturated, monosaturated and saturated, though no fat is wholly one type. Butter, for example, contains 40 per cent saturated and 4 per cent polyunsaturated fat. The health warnings primarily concern saturated fats, which are difficult for the body to absorb and are believed to increase cholesterol levels and cause the arteries to block up. Monosaturates are believed to have a neutral effect on cholesterol and polyunsaturates to keep the cholesterol level low. Only 25 per cent of the cholesterol in the body comes, however, directly from what you eat; the rest is made within the body.

Despite official warnings and the fact that 31 per cent of men and 23 per cent of women in Britain die of heart disease, the message concerning fat intake has been slow to filter through to the public. We are eating roughly the same amount of saturated fat now as we were 20 years ago – before aerobics, mass marathons and a presumed heightened public awareness of health. Yet it is not particularly difficult to overcome the potential disaster of taking on board too much fat. As the Department of Health's COMA report states: "About 40 per cent of the decreases in saturated fatty acids and fat recommended nationally could be achieved by avoiding cream, replacing whole milk with semi-skimmed milk and switching to lower fat cheeses. If skimmed milk was used, approximately 80 per cent of the decreases recommended nationally would be accomplished."

Even if that does not get through to you, and the idea of eating margarine rather than butter is abhorrent, consider also that fat has a high calorific content. When you smear your toast with butter, remember that one ounce of this saturated fat is equivalent to half a pound of potatoes, a complex carbohydrate. Fats contain nine calories per gram and complex carbohydrates four calories per gram, so that you can eat nearly double the amount of carbohydrates to fats for the same amount of energy. It is the butter, cream and bolognese sauce that put on the pounds, not the bread, potatoes and pasta, so if you want to encourage weight loss, cut down your overall fat consumption.

The fat in food

Meat	percentage fat	Cheese	
Fried streaky bacon	45%	Cream cheeses	50%
Grilled streaky bacon	36%	Stilton	40%
Grilled lamb chops	29%	Cheddar	34%
Pork pie	27%	Parmesan	30%
Luncheon meat	27%	Processed cheese	25%
Liver sausage	27%	Camembert	23%
Roast lamb (shoulder)	26%	Edam	23%
Fried pork sausages	25%	Cheese spread	23%
Roast leg of pork	20%	Cottage cheese	4%
Fried beefburgers	17%		
Grilled rump steak	12%	**Milk, butter, oils**	
Casseroled pig's liver	8%	Oil (all kinds)	100%
Stewed steak	7%	Lard	99%
Casseroled chicken	7%	Butter	82%
Fried lamb's kidneys	6%	Margarine (all kinds)	80%
Tinned ham	5%	Double cream	50%
		Dairy ice-cream	7%
Fish		Gold-top milk	5%
Smoked mackerel	16%	Silver-top milk	4%
Fried fish fingers	13%	Yoghurt	1%
Grilled kippers	12%	Skimmed milk	Less than 1%
Cod fried in batter	10%		
Steamed plaice	2%		
Steamed haddock	1%		

One difficulty about cutting down on saturated fats in favour of polyunsaturated fats is distinguishing between them. In general, saturated fats tend to be hard at room temperature – lard and butter, for example – whereas polyunsaturated fats tend to be oily – soft margarine. Exceptions are coconut or palm oils, which are saturated fats. The list on the right gives a guide to the three types of fat found in common food, and the tables show the percentages of fat and saturated fat in commonly consumed foods.

The types of fat in food

Saturated
Beef, lamb, pork, bacon, sausages, salami, fat on meat, meat dripping, lard, butter, ice-cream (some), whole milk, cheese, cream, hard margarines, pastry shortening, coconut oil.

Polyunsaturated
Fish, fish oil, soft margarines, soya beans, most oils – soya, sesame, safflower, sunflower, corn, wheatgerm, cottonseed.

Monosaturated
Chicken, turkey, duck, goose, game, nuts, olive oil, peanut oil.

The saturated fat in fatty food

These figures show the percentage of saturated fat in the total fat content of the food we eat, for example full cream milk (gold-top) is 5% fat. Two thirds (60%) of that fat is saturated.

All dairy products
Milk   about 60%
Butter
Cheese
Cream

Margarines
hard (in packets)   about 40%

soft (in tubs)
   typical blends   about 30%

   "high in
   polyunsaturates"   about 20%

Fats and oils
Coconut oil   about 75%

Lard   about 45%

Blended cooking fat   about 40%

Corn oil   about 20%
Groundnut (peanut) oil
Olive oil
Soya oil

Sunflower oil   less than 15%
Safflower oil

Meats
Lamb fat   about 50%

Beef fat   about 45%

Pork fat   about 40%

Chicken fat   about 35%

Fish
Mackerel   about 25%
Cod
Plaice

Herring   about 20%

How to cut out excess fat in your diet

- Switch to low-fat dairy products.
- Boil or grill rather than fry foods.
- If roasting, place joints on a grill so that fat drains off.
- If frying, use a non-stick pan and spray oil on to the surface (or wipe it on with a paper cloth); use a polyunsaturated oil.
- Pierce sausages thoroughly before cooking and afterwards use kitchen paper to absorb excess fat.
- Brush meats with stock rather than oil if they are to be grilled.
- Remove skin from meat; most of the fat in meat is in the skin.
- Prepare casseroles in advance. Allow to cool and remove fat that has risen to the top before re-heating.
- Use as little butter as possible for cooking.
- Eat water-packed not oil-packed fish.
- If you do use cream, make it single rather than double cream.
- Use soft margarine high in polyunsaturates; avoid products labelled blended vegetable oils (they are normally made from palm and coconut oils).

Carbohydrates

There are two types of carbohydrates: simple and complex. The first is the one with which we are probably most familiar and the one that we should try to avoid. It is sugar, and is commonly referred to as "refined" carbohydrate because it is refined from sugar cane or beet. There is no nutritional value in simple carbohydrates, although the body easily absorbs sugar to give a quick rise in blood glucose levels and hence an "energy lift". Apart from the taste, this is why we tend to eat sugar, although in fact glucose is present in other foods and there is no necessity to resort to sweets, cakes and biscuits – the main forms in which we eat sugar, apart from the white sugar (sucrose) that we might put in our tea or coffee.

Sugar not only contributes nothing to good health but it is also a major reason for excess body fat. We are born with a certain amount of fat cells, which can multiply dramatically in childhood if our diets are high in sugars and fatty foods. In adulthood, fat cells no longer multiply, they simply enlarge and in some people seem to have an almost infinite capacity to do so. Even if you rebalance your weight through sound nutrition and exercise, these "fat" cells do not disappear, they shrink.

The Health Education Council recommends that as a nation we should cut our sugar consumption by half. This is obviously wise advice, both for health and appearance, and although it is not possible to eliminate sugar from your diet completely, you should try to steer clear of it during the 12-week course – and afterwards. The obvious things to avoid are chocolate and other sweets, cakes, biscuits and puddings, but remember that many soft and hard drinks (see alcohol section) contain high levels of sugar. Also, the fact that not all sugars are equally sweet does not mean that the effect on the body is different. And do not be fooled that honey is somehow an exception; it is sugar.

Complex carbohydrates, on the other hand, are important for a well-balanced diet. These are found in vegetables, fruits, pulses and grains. You can get all the energy that you need and even your sweeteners from complex carbohydrates. Moreover, the glucose found in fruit and vegetables does not tax the body in the same way as if taken in simple carbohydrate form, nor

How to cut out excess sugar in your diet

- Use artificial sweeteners in tea or coffee (but aim to stop using these too).
- Eliminate or at least cut down consumption of sweets, biscuits, cakes, pastries and sweet puddings.
- Avoid processed foods that show a high sugar content on the label; try "reduced sugar" jams and marmalades.
- Drink low-calorie soft drinks and fruit juices rather than squashes, but check that fruit juices do not contain sugar. If possible, buy fresh fruit and squeeze it yourself.
- Try apple or pear concentrate (available from health food shops) as a sweetener.
- Squeeze orange juice over fruit to sweeten it instead of sugar.
- Use less sugar when cooking; recipes frequently cater for sweet tooths and the amount can be cut down or an artificial sweetener substituted.
- Buy sugarless muesli and use dried fruits to sweeten it – but make sure that the fruits are not preserved in glucose (normal in supermarkets).
- Eat natural yoghurt rather than fruit yoghurt; the latter has a higher sugar content.
- Have fresh or stewed fruit for pudding.
- Avoid alcohol with a high sugar content, such as beer (see alcohol section).

leave you hungry as quickly because they contain fibre, which takes longer to metabolise. The arguments in favour of eating more complex carbohydrates rather than meat and in place of sugar are well founded and it is advised that during your 12-week course, you aim to establish a diet with a good balance of foods containing them.

Complex carbohydrate foods

Grains – *wheat, oats, corn, rice*

Pasta – *macaroni, spaghetti, noodles, etc.*

Breads

Cereals

Root vegetables – *potatoes, etc.*

Beans and pulses

Most people must by now be aware of the fibre theory and know that it is considered an essential element of diet even if it is basically indigestible. It is now thought better to obtain fibre naturally from foods than to eat a spoonful of bran every day.

High-fibre foods

Wholemeal bread

Brown rice

Potatoes (with jackets), peas, beans

Fruits

Nuts

Cereals

Salt

Salt is a habit. Many people do not believe that food can be tasty without it, whatever cookery experts may say and whatever harm it may do to unseen arteries. Whether you cook with lashings of it, or none at all, it is almost guaranteed that at table hands will reach out for the salt cellar – even before the food has been tasted. In fact salt is naturally available in meat, fish, vegetables, grains and fruits, and food need not be bland if

no more salt is added. If necessary, flavour can be brought out by using herbs and spices, without any risk of causing blood pressure problems.

During the programme to shape up, it is worth trying to cut down salt consumption. Most of the excess comes from an over-liberal hand with the salt cellar and from eating salted crisps or nuts and such processed foods as bacon, sausages, cheese and tinned vegetables. On average, we consume 12 grams of salt a day; to reduce this by half is beneficial even for the physically active, and it should not be difficult.

How to cut out excess salt in your diet

- Avoid nibbling crisps and salted nuts.
- Cut down on processed foods with a high salt content (cured meats, sausages, cheese).
- Taste food before adding salt.
- Season dishes with herbs and spices.
- Use table salt substitutes, such as ruthmol (a low-sodium salt rich in potassium) or miso (a flavouring substance produced from cereals).

Coffee

If you are a heavy coffee drinker, this is a good time to try to reduce your intake. Coffee has no nutritional value and can cause imbibers palpitations, dizziness and insomnia. Purists would have you cut out the habit completely but if you are a "God, I need a cup of coffee to keep going" type, try at least to restrict yourself to three average-size cups a day. It is above this level that the jitters are liable to start.

To help you cut down, drink de-caffeinated instant coffee, or try de-caffeinated coffee beans. Dandelion coffee (available from health food shops) tends to be an acquired taste but you might consider trying it or one of the wealth of herb teas on the market. You will probably either love them or hate them. Consider also cold drinks – low-calorie soft drinks, fruit juices, mineral water or just plain water.

Alcohol

"Alcohol should not be considered as part of the normal diet. To do so implies that it is a necessary component of normal life." However correct these words from the Health Education Council, most men and an increasing number of women find that alcohol is very much part of their normal lives, an accepted way of helping along business deals, enhancing celebrations, unwinding after a pressured day and easing social and work relations generally. Nevertheless, there is no doubt of the harmful effects of excessive alcohol consumption and the 12-week programme is the time to take stock of your drinking habits.

The effect of alcohol depends to a large extent on your body size – a large man is generally able to tolerate more than a small man, and men in general more than women. It also depends on the speed at which you drink and whether you eat when drinking, as well of course as on the current state of your liver. Alcohol does, however, always have some effect on the body and the more accustomed you are to drinking, the less noticeable the outward signs of overconsumption. A man who has drunk 1½ pints of beer (or three shorts) may simply feel increased cheerfulness and to an untrained eye seem very good-natured, but there is always a loss of

---

❝The great American foodie, James Beard, once observed: *'A gourmet who thinks of calories is like a tart who looks at her watch.'* I agree. Foodies are concerned about one thing – taste. Cost, inconvenience, time and patience are but minor considerations, overshadowed by the final result which must excite the eye and delight the palate. So how does a gourmet tackle a three-month regime dedicated to getting him back in shape?

One looks to the French for inspiration. Although on the whole they are an unhealthy lot – gasping on Gitanes all day long and succumbing to cirrhosis of the liver – some of their leading chefs have begun to take a look at the way they cook their food. The days of Escoffier are over and with it the tradition that everything must be cooked in butter and cream. Now we have the clever Michel Guerard, who realised that the emphasis was turning to health and devised *cuisine minceur* to meet the demands of the guests at his wife's spa hotel in the south of France. There are lessons to be learned from this method but through it I came to realise that I could still eat a decent meal and not feel that for 12 weeks I was destined to stick to undressed salads and yoghurts.

Denial is a tricky thing. It was important, given that I had put myself forward as a guinea-pig (is it true that they make good eating?), that I should make a few ground rules for myself. There was no point banning everything because I would be back eating it before long. Did you know that the demand for Mars bars is extremely heavy in villages that are in close proximity to health farms? Denial equals desire.

Of course it was clear to me that I must be as disciplined on the track as when propping up a bar or contemplating a menu. I was told firmly, *'It's no use you doing all this exercise if you are going to go and ruin it all by eating silly food all the time.'*

'Silly food – my goodness, what is that?' I wondered. *'Jellies in the shape of bosoms adorned with marching cherries?'*

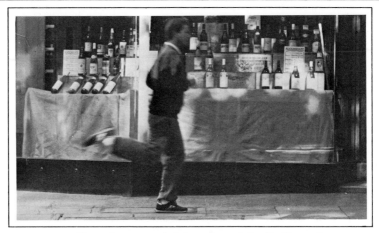

"I put from my mind the talent of the distiller and the brewer – at least for the most part."

'Don't be facetious. You know well enough – stupidly fattening food, dead food, food with empty calories . . .'

Thus, for the most part, I put from my mind delicious cheese boards representing the skill of *fromagers* from dusty corners of France, the art of the *pâtissier* and the *saucier* – and to a great extent the talent of the distiller and brewer. Oh, sad days – but it was not to be just One-Cal Coke existence. Like Gandhi and his virgins, I stepped resolutely into my favourite restaurants, determined to test my will power against the skill of the chef. Sometimes it was a hard battle and sometimes I didn't win.

Imagine the astonishment of one lunchtime companion, whom I had been boring through the starter and the main course about my three-month plan, when for the third course I ordered Prince Charles's own favourite nursery dish, bread and butter pudding. Yes, I know that it contains butter, sugar, eggs, dried fruit and bread – but the image of pudding had been haunting my mind for days and at times I could taste it. To prevent further punishment, I selected, ate and enjoyed a very passable bread and butter pudding. *Result:* no more vivid images of the dish impinged upon my consciousness. I was cured.

My job demanded that I socialise – so socialise I did. That meant still going to the pub, still having business lunches and still attending champagne receptions. Besides, it was not my style to sit alone in an empty office over lunch with a cottage cheese roll, a low fat yoghurt, a low calorie Coca-Cola and a Cox's Orange Pippin for company. I lived out the regime in public, and to some extent concealed it from colleagues, who didn't always refrain from attempting to persuade me back to my old ways.**"**

Neil

judgement. On five pints of beer (10 shorts) this convivial man may turn extremely aggressive and over-exuberant – and he is 25 times more likely to be involved in a road accident.

The Royal College of Physicians recommends that men should not consume more than four pints of beer (8 shorts) on any day – a generous allowance – with at least two consecutive non-drinking days per week, but it also points out that a mere 20g of alcohol a day (equivalent to one pint of beer) is the safest level.

Apart from what alcohol does to your mental, physical and emotional well-being, it also tends to affect your girth: alcohol has a high sugar content. For all these reasons, it is advisable to watch your alcohol consumption level and, if you are a heavy drinker, to reduce it dramatically. During the shape-up programme, follow the guidelines below.

Drinking guidelines

● Give your liver a break. If you must imbibe, drink wine not beer or spirits, and make it a rule to drink no more than three glasses of wine a day.

● Dilute your drinks, which will help cut down on sugar as well as alcohol consumption provided that you do not use sweet mixers. Try soda or mineral water instead.

● Drink a glass of water or fruit juice before you start on alcohol if you are thirsty.

● Intersperse alcoholic drinks with soft, low-calorie drinks or fruit juice.

● Eat something when you drink, which helps to prevent dangerously high levels of alcohol in the blood.

● Get your excuses ready to combat the heavy social pressure to drink; for example, you might try "Had too much last night" or "Doctor's orders" or "On antibiotics".

● Choose a non-alcoholic drink that looks alcoholic to avoid questioning and look part of the drinking company: tonic water (slimline) with a slice of lemon for gin and tonic; ginger ale (slimline) for whisky or brandy; mineral water with angostura bitters for fizzy pink gin; orange juice for vodka and orange; tomato juice – Virgin Mary – for Bloody Mary.

Smoking

Although tobacco is not of course a food or drink, it is often associated with drinking and mealtimes and there is no better time to try to give up smoking than during the programme because getting fit makes giving up easier.

The facts about smoking have undoubtedly reached the public, and over a million people gave up the habit between 1980 and 1982. Most smokers are well aware that they are twice as likely to die of coronary attacks than non-smokers and that smoking is a chief cause of lung cancer and chest diseases. Most smokers also tend to know a relation or friend who smoked 40 cigarettes a day till they died happily at 90. Smoking is like gambling: it may be stimulating and pleasurable but frequently the house wins and the gambler is left poorer if not bankrupt.

One of the most depressing aspects of giving up smoking is the tendency to put on weight, especially during the first year. Remember, however, that vigorous exercise helps reduce appetite and to control weight gain. There is even a theory that it may do more than this to help smokers. Geoffrey Cannon, co-author of *Dieting Makes You Fat*, reports that half the smokers in running groups that he was involved with gave up smoking. The latest explanation for this is that nicotine inhibits the natural flow of endorphins – an artificial substance that acts like an opiate on the body – and creates an artificial substitute for them. During vigorous exercise, the natural endorphin levels are supposed to increase, so that smokers who take up running feel less need for nicotine. Conservative opinion is unconvinced by this theory, and reckons that you would have to be running at least 10 miles each session to obtain the effect. But even if the theory is debatable, vigorous exercise will undoubtedly increase the efficiency of your lungs and be an incentive to stop smoking.

"America, it has been claimed, is turning away from alcohol. While to be seen drinking a dry, very dry, martini in the lounge of the Algonquin might not have the same social cachet as when Dorothy Parker was in residence, a recent survey for *Time* magazine revealed that 67 per cent of adult Americans admitted to drinking. Cynics might suggest that the total is much higher than this because heavy drinkers and alcoholics do not like to go down as drinkers. In Britain, where perhaps we are a more honest lot, statistics show that 95 per cent of all adults take a drink.

Don't think that they are not a dissolute lot in the States. What they are is body-conscious. Apparently it is now OK for chaps to order a light beer without completely losing their manhood. *'There's a reverse psychology at work,'* says one American social watcher, *'you're going to be fat and unattractive if you don't order it. Looking good is the very key.'* The humorist, Fran Lebowitz, has a more down-to-earth view of this abstemiousness. *'It's all part of a wave of self-love. They've overweighted the sanctity of the human body. These bodies aren't temples. They're barely bodegas.'*

Man's desire to be different has given birth to the mineral water snob. If we are no longer allowed to show off our knowledge of wine, we can at least display enormous pretension in the field of H_2O. Thus – Perrier is just a drink for starlets, ice should be left out as it 'bruises the bubbles' and San Pellegrino has a 'springwater flavour, is balanced and sprightly'.

I wasn't going to follow the new American fashion, even if I could. I continued to drink, but in reduced quantities – and it had nothing to do with a somewhat frightening report listing those professions that are more at risk from cirrhosis. Journalist was inevitably well placed, alongside as a matter of interest doctors (hypocrites), army personnel, fishermen and seamen (out of boredom?), garage proprietors (explain that if you can), bar staff, restaurateurs and publicans (top of the list).

I banned beer from my plan because of its heavy content of sugar, and whenever I walked into a pub, I reminded myself that I was in the middle of a programme designed to get me into shape. From time to time little pictures formed in my mind of frothing pints of ale and dripping tankards of lager. I remained strong and emptied these visions down the sink.

The Spritzer was my answer. It is a refreshing mix of dry white wine plus soda or mineral water with a slice of lemon and ice. As the weather got warmer, the drink became more suitable. It's long, tasty, and not too fattening. I allowed myself three a day. As the official figures reveal, I lost over a stone in the three-month period. And it was almost painless. I continued to eat well and never felt hungry, and I was still able to enjoy a drink.**"**

Neil

Surviving the Hazards of Eating Out

General rules

Eschew

aperitifs

olives/salted nuts

rolls and butter

liqueurs

puddings/cheese

Go for

mineral water instead

gherkins/onions/unroasted nuts

dry bread sticks if you must

coffee without cream and sugar
   (use saccharine)

fresh fruit

"Mouth watering, I visualise the ticks and crosses against the delights on this menu, and no, I didn't have to keep to undressed salads and sticks of celery. I would choose only creations prepared without cream or butter – delicious, and designed not to terminate life prematurely."

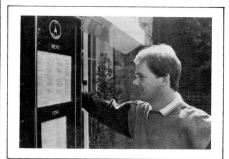

Pub Menu

Crisps ✗✗✗

Dry roasted or salted peanuts ✗✗✗

Soup ✓✓✓

Pâté and bread ✓✓✓

Mackerel pâté ✓✓

Wholemeal bread sandwiches ✓✓✓

Welsh rarebit ✗

Ploughman's lunch ✗✗

Scotch eggs ✗

Veal and ham pie ✓

Cornish pasty ✓

Pub curries ✓

Steak and kidney pie ✓

Pork pie ✗✗

Fish pie ✓✓

Hamburger, chips and beans ✗✗

Slice of pizza ✓✓

Chilli con carne ✓

Sausage and chips ✗✗

Cold meats and salad ✓✓

Plaice and chips ✓

Scampi in a basket ✗

Chicken pie and peas ✓✓

Jellied eels ✓✓✓

Chicken, turkey, beef and ham salads ✓✓

Baked potatoes with sour cream ✓✓✓

Baked potatoes with chilli stuffing ✓

Lasagne ✗

Quiche ✓

Smoked trout with horseradish ✓✓✓

Devilled whitebait ✗

Veal chops (grilled) ✓

Steak, chips and salad ✗✗

Shepherd's pie ✓

Restaurant Menu

STARTERS

Melon with ginger ✓✓✓✓
Melon with fresh fruit ✓✓✓
Melon and Parma ham ✓
Avocado vinaigrette ✗
Avocado prawns ✗
Prawn cocktail ✗
Chicken liver pâté ✓
Kipper pâté ✓✓
Duck pâté ✗
Cream of mushroom soup ✓
Lentil and orange soup ✓✓✓
Crudités ✓✓✓
Salad of artichoke and prawns ✓✓✓
Seafood salad ✓✓
Clam fries ✗✗
Mediterranean prawns ✓✓✓
Deep fried Camembert ✗✗✗
Whitebait ✗
Grilled sardines ✓✓✓
Potted shrimps ✗
Smoked salmon ✓
Salmon mousse ✓
Arbroath smokie mousse with smoked salmon ✓

FISH

Trout with almonds ✓
Trout with Hollandaise sauce ✓✓
Whole poached salmon ✓✓✓
Fried scallops ✗✗
Scallops Mornay in white wine and cheese sauce ✗
Scampi Meunière ✓
Scampi Provençale poached in tomato sauce ✓✓✓
Scampi Maison – deep fried with tartare sauce ✗✗
Sole grilled ✓✓✓
Sole Bonne Femme – served with mushrooms,
onions and parsley sauce ✓✓
Sole Mornay, glazed with cheese sauce ✗✗
Sole Colbert – deep fried ✗✗✗
Pan-fried halibut ✗
Grilled, skewered monkfish ✓✓✓
Turbot, grilled ✓✓✓
Turbot in white wine sauce ✓

MEAT

Roast chicken ✓✓✓
Chicken brochette ✓✓
Breast of chicken stuffed with truffles ✓✓
Chicken in barbecue sauce ✓✓
Chicken and mushroom pie ✓
Chicken Kiev ✗✗✗
Chicken in puff pastry stuffed with ham, cream
and mushrooms ✗✗✗
Veal in cream and tarragon sauce ✗
Roast veal with red wine and rosemary sauce ✓✓
Calves liver with onions and bacon ✗✗
Grilled pork chops with apple sauce ✓
Grilled Scotch sirloin with Bearnaise sauce ✗
Peppered steak ✗
Fillet steak grilled with salad ✓
Rack of lamb ✓
Loin of lamb rosettes pan-fried and served in port ✗✗
Roast leg of lamb, roast potatoes and vegetables of
the day ✓
Roast beef with vegetables of the day and roast
potatoes ✓
Beef Wellington, cooked with pâté and wrapped in
pastry ✗✗
Mixed grill with chips ✗
Breast of duck sautéd in butter and Calvados ✗
Crispy roasted duckling ✓

SALADS

Turkey salad ✓✓✓
Tuna salad ✓✓✓
Chef's salad ✓✓
Chicken and ham salad ✓✓
Roast beef salad ✓✓
Oyster salad ✓✓✓
Prawn, crab or lobster salad ✓✓✓
Mixed salad with slices of foie gras ✓✓

DESSERTS

Sweets from the trolley ✗✗✗
Fresh fruit ✓✓✓
Fruit salad ✓
Cheese board ✗✗✗

Chinese Menu

Barbecued pork spare ribs ✗
Fried seaweed ✓
Deep fried prawn balls ✗✗
Spring rolls ✗
Grilled dumplings ✓✓✓ ✓✓✓
Crabmeat and sweetcorn soup ✓✓✓
Hot and sour soup ✓✓ ✓✓✓
Fresh prawn wan tun ✓✓✓

Aromatic crispy lamb ✓✓✓
Steamed fish, whole ✓✓✓
Fresh crab with ginger and spring onions ✓✓
Grilled prawns Peking-style ✓✓✓
Prawns in sweet and sour sauce ✗
Quick fried prawns with green peppers ✗
Barbecued Peking duck ✓✓
Diced chicken with cashew nuts and yellow
bean sauce ✓
Chicken Peking-style ✓✓✓
Sweet and sour pork ✗✗✗
Grilled pork Peking-style ✓
Fried beef with black bean sauce ✗✗✗
Quick fried lamb with spring onions ✗✗✗

Fresh Chinese vegetables ✓✓✓
Fresh beans with garlic ✓✓✓
Beanshoots ✓✓✓
Grilled or steamed dumplings ✓✓✓
Special fried rice ✗✗
Steamed rice ✓✓✓

Greek Menu

STARTERS
Egg and lemon soup (avgolemono) ✓✓✓
Aubergine fritters (melitzanes tiryanites) ✗✗
Stuffed tomatoes (domates yemistes) ✓✓✓
Dolmathes (stuffed vine leaf with mince) ✓✓
Taramasalata (cod's roe) ✓✓
Hummus (chick peas) ✓✓✓
Pitta bread ✓✓✓
Fried triangles of flaky pastry filled with
minced lamb (kreatopitta) ✗✗✗
Fried triangles of flaky pastry filled with
fetta cheese and herbs (tigropitta) ✗✗
Greek salad (feta cheese, tomatoes,
onions, olives) ✓✓✓

MAIN COURSES
Stuffed aubergines (melitzanes
yemistes) ✓✓
Moussaka ✗
Meat balls in egg and lemon sauce
(youvarlakia)
Roast lamb (arni pasto) ✓✓
Lamb fricassee with egg and lemon
sauce (arni fricasse avgolemono) ✗
Shish kebab (arni souvlakia) ✓✓✓
Fat spiced meat balls (grilled sheffalia) ✗✗✗
Dry stew with onions and coriander
seeds (pork afelia) ✗✗
Suckling pig stuffed with feta
(gourounaki yemisto me feta) ✗✗✗
Fried fish with sauce (psari me saltsa) ✗✗
Grilled fish (psito psari) ✓✓✓
Squid fried in oil and garlic (calamares) ✗✗

Greek coffee
plain ✓   sweet ✗✗✗

Indian Menu

Papadum (fried) ✗✗✗
Papadum (roasted) ✓
Onion bhajee ✗✗✗
Mulligatawny soup ✓
Dall soup ✓✓

Chicken tikka ✓✓✓
Lamb tikka ✓
Tandoori mixed grill ✓
Tandoori lobster (king sized prawns) ✓✓✓
Chicken curry ✓
Ceylon chicken curry ✓✓
Tandoori butter chicken ✗✗✗
Chicken pulau ✓✓✓
Prawn korma ✓
Tandoori fish masala ✓✓✓
Vegetable biryani ✓✓✓
Chicken biryani ✓✓✓
Prawn biryani ✓✓✓
Vegetable curry ✓✓✓
Matter panner ✓

Raita ✓✓✓
Plain rice ✓✓✓
Pulao rice ✓✓✓
Chapati ✓✓✓
Nan plain ✓✓
Keema nan ✗

Cheap and Cheerful

Porridge (without sugar) ✓✓✓
Grapefruit (tinned) ✓✓✓
Cornflakes ✗✗
Fried eggs, bacon, tomato, on fried bread ✗✗✗
Eggs, bacon, beans on toast ✗
Beans on toast ✓✓
Poached eggs ✓✓✓
Scrambled eggs ✓✓
Kippers ✓✓✓
Cheese omelette ✓
Sausages and mash ✗
Spaghetti (tinned) on toast ✓✓
Mixed grill ✗
Steak, chips and peas ✗✗
Fried gammon steaks ✗✗
Fish cakes ✓
Toast, marmalade and butter ✓
Bread and jam ✓

"I emptied visions of frothing pints of ale down the sink and kept to wine and mineral water. I lost over a stone in the three-month period."

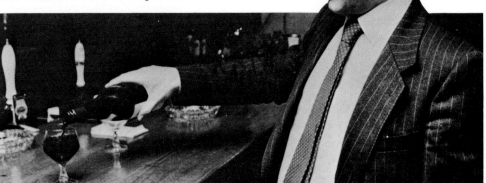

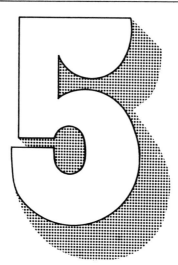

The New Man

WHAT HAPPENS AT THE END of the 12-week plan? The chances are that the new man will have no wish to see his paunch reflate, the early morning tiredness descend again and his new-found energy dissipate. If he now wants to enjoy his old pleasures with moderation, the fitness level that he has achieved will not be dramatically affected for at least a month. Whenever the feeling of well-being begins to fade, the programme can be repeated to recapture it. He may wish to make it a regular part of his life, or to achieve greater fitness by moving on to a more advanced level. Whatever the decision, the key is enjoyment.

I have to admit that I never thought Neil would make it. I didn't think that I could counteract the lure of Fleet Street; even though the scheme was tailor-made for him, I was sure that one of his fellow hacks would sow a seed of doubt into the 'ridiculous' new life-style that he was adopting. But surprise, surprise, one or two of these hardened hacks soon began to make complimentary remarks to me about Neil. I didn't hear the usual scorn in their voices for the cause of fitness. Other friends were even more enthusiastic. One told me, 'You must make sure that Neil keeps on with this. He really is a different man.'

It was true, but would it last? I was thrilled to have back the man I had married, who was less tired, easier-going and generally more active! But could he sustain it? What has happened since the end of the programme is that when he has a major lapse into unfitness, he actually wants to do something about it, to shape up again. The 12-week course had given him a point of comparison – what it feels like to be fit.

To me the highlight of the whole programme was not simply that he was more active but that psychologically he was so different. He seemed more on top of life, able to cope with the daily hassles. He was more relaxed, confident and positive. It was worth all the effort that I put into the 12 weeks to have my man back.

Catherine

❝During a convivial lunch the other day with two colleagues, we got to that stage of the meal when brandies are swirled in the warming palm of the hand and we started to reflect on our general good fortune. It was exactly occasions like these, we agreed, that made life bearable. But then one of my colleagues, remembering that I was involved in this book, turned to me accusingly, 'But of course *you* want to put a stop to all this.'

It was an unfair accusation. At the outset of this project I might have had a similar response to a friend who was apparently coming over all-Puritan and wanting to denounce the good things in life – drink, restaurant meals, late nights, fish and chips, or whatever. I still believe in the long lunch, the joys of claret, the delights of a creatively cooked French meal followed by at least two fine brandies.

The difference now is that I have had a peek – a retrospective peek – at how it was to be aged 25. That was 10 years ago and in the fog of my mind I can still remember playing three sets of tennis and not feeling anything other than a little relaxed. As I have admitted, when I began this course I could only manage to run for about eight minutes before feeling that my lungs were filling up with some liquid akin to Brasso. At the end of the 12 weeks – and here I want to boast – I could run for an hour or so, with enjoyment.

As the course came to its conclusion, I noticed that the bulge, once as immovable as Mount Idris, had actually gone to Mohammed. It was not that I needed my trousers taking in – I had always been vain enough to stick to a size 32-inch waist despite the progress of the pot. It meant that I looked better – and I not only have my wife's testimony to this point but the unbiased words of mere acquaintances, who suggested that a certain youthful bloom had returned to my cheeks. Requests for the miracle diet that I was clearly on were made, and never met – because I was never on a diet.

Certainly I was less tired during the day. Most probably I slept better. I didn't miss the hangovers and I still enjoyed the lunches. The physical exhilaration of dashing through a park as the sluggish loafed around walking their poodles was wonderful. When you are flying along, anything seems possible.

After all the work I have put in pounding the pavements, I think that I can safely promise that it is all worthwhile. I don't expect to live longer, to grey later and to show a superb improvement in bed; but I know I don't wish to return to that point of grubby wretchedness that I had reached before I began this whole plan. If the inches creep back around the stomach and the heaviness and the slothfulness return, I will remember how I was after I had tuned up for three months. It will be, is, a nice feeling.

There's nothing cissy about getting shaped up, although those who try to take stock of their expanding personal assets may be accused of reaching the male menopause, being frightened of death, or of being quite simply boring and a killjoy. Their accusers will be in the unhappy position of failing to take the responsibility for their own well-being. As Dr Johnson, a man who was no stranger to the pub, said: 'I look upon it that he who does not mind his belly will hardly mind anything else.'**❞**

The Birmingham Report

THE THREE TESTS PERFORMED were for aerobic capacity, including lung function, leg power and body fat. These are the main areas in which the recreational exerciser generally wants to improve. The first concerns the ability of the lungs, heart and blood system to deliver oxygen to the working muscles, and also the ability of the muscles themselves to use this extra oxygen; the second is about muscle speed and power – many exercisers want to become a little faster; and the third is about body fat – very many exercisers want to lose fat, which they may often inaccurately describe as wanting to lose weight.

Aerobic capacity

This test was performed on a treadmill, and the exercise level was designed to bring the subject up to the range of his age-related heart rate (in Neil's case 187 at 33 years old). The respiratory measures were made with an "Oxycon" automated analysis system, with Neil wearing a face mask with a nose-clip. His heart rate was measured by surface chest electrodes, which gave both a visual display and a direct recording on the Oxycon print-out. The results were as follows:

	First test	Second test (3 months later)
Length of test	8 min 15 sec	9 min
Final speed	9 mph	10 mph
Maximum ventilation	113.4 litres/min	97.7 litres/min
Oxygen uptake	47.1 ml/kg	48.7 ml/kg
Respiratory quotient	1.00 at 6 min, heart rate of 186; 1.07 at end, heart rate of 194	0.92 at 6 min, heart rate of 170; 0.96 at end, heart rate of 182
Maximum heart rate	194	182
Oxygen debt	6.44 litres (87 ml/kg)	3.83 litres (56 ml/kg)

COMMENTS: On his first visit, Neil ran 3 minutes at 6 mph and 3 at 8 mph; then, because his heart rate had reached 186, the speed was set at 9 rather than 10 mph, at which he ran 2 minutes 15 seconds before stopping. On his second visit, he not only completed the 9 minutes of the test but was able to run the final 3 minutes at a speed of 10 mph.

The drop in maximum ventilation from 113.4 litres per minute at the end of the first test to 97.7 litres per minute at the end of the second – longer and harder – test represents a considerable improvement in breathing: on the first test Neil needed to breathe 33.2 ml of air to extract 1.0 ml of oxygen, but on the second test he needed only 30.0 ml of air to extract the same amount of oxygen.

The oxygen uptake of 47.1 ml/kg on the first test was a maximal figure and was in fact reasonably good – about 10 per cent above average normal values. The figure of 48.7 on the second test does not indicate the full extent of Neil's improvement because it was reached at a heart rate of 182, below the maximal rate; his maximum oxygen uptake figure would have been about 52 ml/kg.

The respiratory quotients – the ratio of carbon dioxide breathed out to oxygen breathed in – show a similar large improvement. On the first test, the ratio reached unity – 1.00 – at only six minutes and at a heart rate of 186 and a treadmill speed of 8 mph, whereas on the second test, which was both longer and faster than the first, the ratio never reached unity and the figure of 0.96 was only recorded in the final minute, and then with a heart rate of 182 and at a speed of 10 mph. This meant that Neil's "anaerobic threshold" had risen considerably: he could make much greater exertions before having to use anaerobic or non-oxygen sources of energy, with their attendant penalty of lactic acid build-up and consequent fatigue.

The maximum heart rate figures are particularly telling. The rate of 194 on the first test is 7 beats higher than the accepted "normal" age-related maximum for a 33-year-old, but on the second test the maximum heart rate reached was only 182, even though the test was 10 per cent harder. The strain on the heart was much less.

On both tests, the oxygen debt figures are good. We did not try to assess on either occasion the near-maximum oxygen debt that Neil would incur, so the figures are not proof of improvement, although clearly the drop to 3.83 litres (56 ml/kg) shows that Neil required a much lower oxygen debt to complete the second test.

Overall, the results show a very significant increase in all aspects of aerobic power as a result of Neil's training programme. This is the more impressive because Neil was rather above average in aerobic fitness to start with, which makes it harder to improve.

Lung function is tested with a spirometer and is mainly intended to motivate smokers and assess asthmatics, neither of which applied to Neil. Provided that the lungs are healthy to begin with, little or no change is expected in the results of tests made before and after an exercise programme. This was true in Neil's case: the "vital capacity" – the volume of air following the biggest inhalation and the biggest exhalation – was 3.96 litres on the first test and 3.91 on the second, an insignificant difference.

It is not the lungs (unless they are affected by smoking, bronchitis, asthma or other difficulty) that limit exercise performance. The trouble is not getting air into the chest and then passing oxygen through into the blood, but oxygen *transport* – not being able to passage enough blood. Efficient oxygen transport depends largely on the heart. Following months of exercise, the volume of blood may rise considerably but it is the heart that undergoes the major change: its walls increase in thickness and hence strength, and its chamber size increases. More blood can be pumped out at each beat and hence the oxygen supply to working muscles is increased. As Neil's results show, this is reflected in better aerobic performance on the treadmill and better oxygen uptake levels.

Leg power

This is tested by asking the subject to perform a vertical jump; a reasonable estimate of power in relation to body weight can then be made using the "Lewis Nomogram". Neil's results were:

	First test	Second test
Jump height	38.1 cm (15 in)	44 cm (17¼ in)
Power estimate	102 kg-m/sec	106 kg-m/sec

COMMENTS: The very marked increase is partly due to Neil's lowered body fat percentage and drop in body weight (see below), and partly due to his increased leg strength and power. He started with an already very good leg power factor, which after training rose to a level that put him in the upper range of physical education students.

Body fat

The standard technique was used for this test, which is to measure the skin thickness at four sites with special calipers; conversion tables then give the fat reading as a percentage of body weight. Neil's results were:

	First test	Second test
Skin folds: biceps	6.5 mm	2.5 mm
triceps	11.9 mm	9.6 mm
sub-scapular	18.5 mm	13.4 mm
supra-iliac	26.2 mm	13.0 mm
Body weight	74 kg (163 lb)	68 kg (150 lb)
Fat mass	16.7 kg	11.2 kg
Percentage body fat	22.5	16.5

COMMENTS: Fat and muscle are the main aspects of body mass that can undergo major changes. After months of exercise it is possible for a person to gain muscle and lose fat without showing much loss in body weight, even though considerable changes in body composition may have occurred. Similarly, it is possible to gain weight while having lost fat, and indeed to lose weight while actually having gained fat, as for example, may happen if a person gives up a strenuous regular sport such as rugby.

Neil's results show, however, a dramatic loss in both fat and body weight. The 5.5 kg drop in fat mass, which accounts for almost all of his 6 kg weight difference, amounts to a substantial loss of adipose tissue, or fat; and he has almost halved his "fat roll" at the waist just above the hip bone (supra-iliac crest). He may feel the cold a little more but this should be more than compensated for by greatly increased exercising ability (not to mention appearance).

Dr Craig Sharp
The Human Motor Performance Laboratory, Birmingham University

Strength and co-ordination

	TEST 1 date 17ᵗʰ March	TEST 2 date 7ᵗʰ June	% change
Name Neil Mackwood.			
1. Calf: toe-ups: stand on one leg, go up and down on the toes **right leg:**	30 secs: 36	50	+39
	60 secs: 56	87	+55
left leg:	30 secs: 38	42	+10
	60 secs: 60	80	+33
2. Alternate leg thrusts: rest on palms, kick each leg in turn straight behind	60 secs: 70	89	+27
3. Hamstring kicks: lie on stomach, kick one heel at a time towards seat **right leg:**	30 secs: 39	35	-10
	60 secs: 72	66	-8
left leg:	30 secs: 38	38	—
	60 secs: 64	67	+5
4. Straight-leg raises: knee straight, lift to 32cm, with 2.5kg weight, touching down to floor from each lift **right leg:**	30 secs: 40	50	+25
	60 secs: 86	101	+17
left leg:	30 secs: 40	50	+25
	60 secs: 78	105	+35
5. Hip abduction: lie on each side in turn, balancing on lower elbow and foot, lifting hips up sideways **right side:**	30 secs: 22	37	+68
left side:	30 secs: 17	41	+141
6. Squats: arms held straight forwards, back as straight as possible	60 secs: 37	46	+24
7. Abdominals: sit-ups lying with knees bent, feet fixed, hands behind head	60 secs: 13	18	+38
8. Dorsal rises: for back extensor muscles, performed on Norsk machine	11	26	+136
9. Shoulder abductors: stand with 1.75kg weight in each hand, lift arms straight out sideways	56	52	-7
10. Press-ups:	60 secs: 16	29	+81
11. Biceps curls: rest arms on two pillows, with 1.75kg weight in each hand, bend elbows to touch hands to shoulders	68	91	+34
12. Balance: on each leg in turn, eyes closed **right leg:**	30 secs	133 secs	+343
left leg:	51 secs	171 secs	+235

The Chiswick Report

Together with the results from your laboratory tests, these tests show a considerable improvement. Without quantifying the percentage improvement on the individual tests, it is obvious from the figures how much your general strength and flexibility have been improved by your training programme.

The shoulder abductor exercise did not improve, but I feel this was an aberration, possibly linked to the queasy stomach you had on the day of the repeat tests. The hamstring kicks did improve, despite the figures, as the re-test was done with shoes on, to give weight-resistance.

Besides the actual improvement in the individual tests, the most striking change is in your overall posture and co-ordination. The exercises looked (and were) difficult for you on the first test. On the second, you were performing them efficiently, with ease. Your movement patterns have definitely benefited from your exercise and fitness programme. This will certainly help your squash performance!

Having made such significant improvements in your fitness, I feel you will be able to maintain your fitness levels, and indeed continue your improvement, by doing a further 12-week spell of training, preferably repeating the course at intervals throughout the year. You do not need to exercise continuously to maintain your fitness, so you can have "rest" phases without fearing a return to your previous level of unfitness. Each time you embark on a further spell of progressive, balanced training, you can look forward to further measurable improvements in your fitness.

Your fat levels, for instance, though dramatically reduced, are still capable of great improvement. Your abdominal strength is still not admirable, and improving the condition of your stomach muscles would certainly help reduce the fat cover in the area.

The other very pleasing aspect of your programme has been your apparent freedom from injury and major illness setbacks. Often, the temptation for the "new exerciser" is to set about the programme with such vigour that illness *and* injury inevitably strike, either separately or together. Your programme balance has clearly been just right, both from the physical, and mental attitude, point of view.

Vivian Grisogono

Flexibility

Name Neil Mackwood

		TEST 1 date 17th March	TEST 2 date 7th June	% change
1. **Forward reach**: in hurdle position, with knee straight, extend hand to toes, sit up, keeping back as straight as possible. Distance - middle finger to great toe	right side:	26 cm	4 cm	+550
	left side:	28 cm	5 cm	+460
2. **Front thigh stretch**: lie on stomach, pull each foot gently towards seat Distance - heel to seat	right side:	5 cm	1 cm	+400
	left side:	4·5 cm	3 cm	+50
3. **Trunk extension**: lie on stomach, push trunk up and back gently, resting on hands and straightening elbows. Keep hips on floor. Distance - floor to notch above breast-bone		38 cm	51 cm	+34

Index